Sarah Roberts lives in Sur... husband Chris and their thr... and Flo. Oscar was di... ...nally with Down syndro... ...en he was around eighteen month... ...an started a blog, *Don't Be Sorry*, to ...ais ...awareness about the condition and offer a raw insight into both the challenges he faces and the many positives. She has always referred to the blog as her online therapy, appreciating how cathartic writing things down and talking out loud, sharing our stories can be. Drawing on her blog, which now has a following of over 48,000 and has won many awards, she published her first book, *For the Love of Oscar*, in 2019, chronicling her family life. She has subsequently become a public speaker and freelance writer focusing on the joys and challenges of raising a child with additional needs.

In creating this blog, Sarah has found herself with a platform to help others either struggling to come to terms with their child's diagnosis or other difficulties. She feels it's a privilege to be contacted by strangers who want to share their stories, their feelings and concerns.

Sarah is now in her second year of training to become a counsellor/psychotherapist and her dream is one day to open her own private practice.

Facebook: dontbesorry2 / Twitter: @dontbesorry2 / Instagram: dontbesorry2

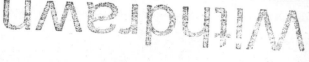

Also by Sarah Roberts

For the Love of Oscar

Contents

Prologue

A message popped into my in-box late one Friday evening. It was the kind of message you get that you read and feel you can't leave to come back to after the weekend. They needed me now. It went something along the lines of this. . .

'I've had a baby two days ago and he has Down's syndrome. I'm struggling so hard. I just don't know who to turn too. Everyone I know is sending me congratulations on my beautiful baby and I just want to scream. I can't manage to think beyond what's happening right now without getting massive anxiety. If I think into the future at all, it makes me feel sick. I know in my mind it will be fine, I just want to know it in my heart. It's coming to terms with a new life, a new normal. It's being ok with a baby that doesn't look like us. How long before I can look at all my friends who've just had babies or who are pregnant at the same time as I was and not feel envious. How long did it take you to start adjusting? Last night was the first night I was able to settle him in the night and I think I felt the first drops of love. It is coming. I know it is.'

As I sat and read every word she'd written, recalling how I'd felt just two days after having had Oscar, a wave of sadness came over me. I'd been there you see. Every single word she'd written resonated with me. Yet here I was now, nine years on, someone who'd lived through the highs and lows of parenting a child with Down syndrome and who understood all too well the difficulties. And yet, whilst I'd also lived through the many heart-bursting, pride-inducing moments that come with having a child like ours, I'd still wondered if now was the right time to tell her the truth?

How did I tell her, that I, too, struggled at first. That for a long, long time following Oscar's diagnosis, it felt like someone had ripped out my heart, so much so that it felt like a physical pain?

How did I tell her that every time I received a 'Congratulations on your beautiful baby boy' card and placed it on my windowsill, I resented the card because this wasn't the way I'd planned our lives to go and I couldn't bear looking at them all lined up there?

How did I tell her that the image I'd had of the older gentleman who happened to have Down syndrome, walking around our village on his own, with dodgy clothes and a bad haircut, talking to himself, was the *only* image I pictured back then and that that had scared me? Could I tell her that?

How did I tell her it took that broken heart of mine some time to heal, too?

Did I tell her that when well-meaning people, who'd had older children with DS themselves, spoke about speech therapy, physiotherapy, portage, EHCPs and goodness knows what else came with this new role, how petrified I'd been and how I'd wanted out from the start?

Did I risk telling her that this 'new normal' others talked of filled me with dread and I couldn't for a second see how we could ever be happy again?

How did I say that for a very long time afterwards, when I heard friends or family members had fallen pregnant, I willed something like this to happen to them too because I didn't want to be the only one. I wanted them to feel everything I had. I didn't want to feel alone. Could I tell her that?

I knew the answer. I knew it would be hard reading, but I had to tell her my truth. Because in doing so, hopefully she wouldn't feel so alone. Or as awful as I'd felt for feeling like I was the only person out there, experiencing such dark, dark thoughts.

So, I would tell her how things had been for me back then, but also how they were now. I would tell her that all this was *my* truth and that I wouldn't and couldn't talk on behalf of every mother out there who'd experienced this, because everyone's story is different. I would tell her that the pain had passed sooner than I'd thought it would. It wasn't a thunderbolt-type epiphany or anything like that; it was just that, over time, I realised I wasn't quite as sad as I'd been the week before or the week before that. I would tell her that, in hindsight, I was glad that we'd received the congratulations cards. For I'd decided that it would have been a very sad time if people had felt they couldn't send them because they'd assumed there was nothing to be celebrated. I was so grateful, and I felt their love and support.

I would tell her that the outdated stereotypes are long gone because, in my mind, Oscar is one of the coolest kids I know. I would tell her that with early intervention and not putting limitations on what we think our kids are capable of, kids and adults with DS are achieving so much more than ever before. The new normal? I would say it's not what I'd imagined it would be in the slightest. If anything, it's opened my eyes to a completely different world, one that I love being a part of. I would tell her that the hurt, the upset, the resentment and the worry have long gone now. And I would tell her that the love came thick and fast once all the other stuff had gone.

The thing is, how could I make that sound credible, without it coming across as too happy-clappy. So many people say, 'He/she's a gift from God,' and, 'Special children are given to special people,' when they talk about children who happen to have DS. That 'you're only sent what you can handle' and that you're 'hashtag blessed' is just not my bag. I don't know that I believe any of it, personally. And, as a side note, how do any of us know how it's all going to pan out? How any of our kids, regardless of diagnosis, are going to end up? None of us know, right?

All too often, you assume life's going one way, then it takes a weird and wonderful turn somewhere else. What I do know is that this is *my* experience, no one else's, and although I know others may have felt some of these same emotions, it won't have been like this for everyone.

So, what *do* I say when someone like this woman contacts me, asking me to throw her a life raft because she feels like, right now, she's sinking?

I say, there isn't a day that goes by that I don't look at Oscar's beautiful face and feel so insanely grateful that he's mine. I say that with more certainty, more clarity than anything I've ever felt before. Because that's *my* hand-on-heart truth.

1

Lockdown Runaway

'They laugh at me because I'm different. I laugh at them because they're all the same'

Unknown

It was the spring of 2020. The UK was in lockdown because of the global Covid-19 pandemic, I was at home with three kids (Oscar, 7; Alfie, 6; and Flo, 4), attempting to home-school them. Chris, my husband, was at home too, but thankfully (and resented on my bitter-and-twisted part) he was able to hide in his 'mancave', his purpose-built office/shed at the end of the garden and busy himself with work, earning a living, but mostly, I assumed, avoiding the carnage unfolding around us all.

I cried to my mum down the phone when I told her we'd taken the decision to take the kids out of school, although it ended up being only three days before the rest of the UK. Oscar was classed as 'vulnerable' because of borderline pulmonary hypertension and the anxiety and worry about whether we should take him out of school to avoid the risk of catching the virus was all-consuming. This meant that our other two children would also be taken out of school as there'd be little point in their staying and running the risk of bringing Covid-19 home. I knew it was the right thing to do for Oscar's health. You'd do anything to protect your children, right? But, quite selfishly, the thought of being home 24/7 with three children, one of whom has additional needs, filled me with horror and dread.

As it turns out, we got through it. The home-schooling part was hit and miss. If I managed to get Oscar to sit down and do a ten-minute activity once a day, that was a win in my book, but the hard part was managing what he was up to, whilst focusing my attention on Alfie and Flo's learning.

It was hot that year, so he spent a lot of time in the garden, jumping in and out the paddling pool. We have bifold doors in our kitchen that open out onto the garden, so although I had a good view of what Oscar was doing, there were times when I'd miss some bit of mischief because my attention was on the other two children.

Like the time he managed to drive his Little Tikes car next to one of our neighbour's fence panels, hoist himself up over it, jump down into their garden and run bare-footed into their house. Chris by this point was in hot pursuit. He had had to abruptly leave a Zoom meeting, telling his team he'd be back but he 'just had to go over the garden fence to get his son'. Oscar had found his way upstairs into the neighbour's spare bedroom and was now waving down at me, with the biggest grin on his face. I could feel my cheeks burn with rage, 'GET DOWN!' I mouthed to him, panicking, that lovely Brenda (our elderly neighbour) would be having kittens. At this stage, in the UK, none of us was allowed into each other's houses for fear of spreading Covid-19, so you can imagine the look of horror on my and eventually Brenda's face when we realised what he'd done. Thankfully, she was suitably lovely about it all.

Another time, there'd been a knock at the door, which turned out be another neighbour, who lived opposite, and a sheepish-looking Oscar standing behind her. Apparently, while I'd been reading with Alfie, he'd managed to locate the key to our front door, open it, head over the road and, bold as brass, knock on their door. By all accounts, our neighbour had seen him walking down her driveway and had been concerned that something had happened to either Chris or me, and that Oscar was coming to alert her. As heroic as that sounded, I told her it was more likely that he was after her sons, whom he'd often seen playing football in the street and wanted to join them.

Then there was the day I realised, having taken my eyes off Oscar for a few moments, that he was now nowhere to be seen. I'd raced out into the garden, my heart in my mouth, knowing he had previous for taking any opportunity to 'break out'. I'd started shouting his name, hoping he'd pop out from somewhere and I could go back to Alfie and his 'place value' (yeah, I have no clue either). Except there was no response. Our garden backs onto five other houses, so at this stage of the game he could have been frankly anywhere. After shouting his name a few more times, I heard a giggle and what sounded like a spring going up and down. 'Oscar, WHERE ARE YOU?' I would recognise that cheeky giggle anywhere. He laughed again, clearly finding it hysterical now. As I walked towards where the noise was coming from and peered over the garden fence, I could see Oscar jumping up and down on our neighbour's trampoline, laughing away to himself. The next issue was how to get him back. Our neighbours have no side access and the only way to get into their garden, is through their house. Knowing that they were being super-cautious because a member of their family was vulnerable,

I knew they wouldn't be happy about me walking through their house, or with their little visitor.

We eventually got him out by holding the fence panel up so Chris could crawl underneath and through their bushes to retrieve him. I think Chris had been mid-call again, so obviously this escapade went down like a lead balloon with him. But seriously, this kid!!!

And it's not just Great Escapes that make us known to our neighbours. There was the time, as I was walking back from the village shop, that I was pulled to one side by another neighbour, who let me know that a pair of pants had ended up in his garden. Which then promoted great discussion between him and his wife about whose pants they were because they'd be too big to be Oscar's but seemed 'far too big to be Sarah's'.

As it turns out they *were* mine. I knew they were mine as soon as they started talking, but I was too embarrassed to claim them, knowing that they'd been my GINORMOUS ones that I'd had out on the drying rack a couple of days beforehand. Can you imagine the mortification?

As I write this, Oscar has just turned nine. I remember when I first had Oscar being told that he would be a 'joy' and would 'light up my world'. And whilst I am not denying that he is, and that he has done, he's also aged me by fifty-plus years; he's the reason I'm going grey and often lies at the root of my ever-increasing stress levels.

Just to take those of you who haven't read my first book, *For the Love of Oscar*, back to the start. Oscar was born on 7 July 2012 after a traumatic birth, but what can only be described as a straightforward pregnancy. Chris and I had been fortunate enough to fall pregnant the month after our honeymoon. When I look back on it with the benefit of hindsight, before the brief discussion with the midwife at my twelve-week scan (when she told me they were screening for Down syndrome, Edward's syndrome and Patau's syndrome), DS hadn't even factored in my thoughts.

When I'd had the screening, Oscar had been classed as at 'low risk' of having DS. I could go on and on about this, but I'll just touch on it for now. The word 'risk' when referring to DS is awful. Thankfully, due to many of our community harping on about it so much and campaigning for change, a lot of the literature used by student midwives has now been amended to use the word 'chance' or 'likelihood', e.g. the 'chance' of your baby having DS is 1 in 10,000, as opposed to the 'risk' of your baby having DS. See? Anyway, the word 'risk' is still bandied about by midwives, consultants and sonographers (women write to me regularly to let me know) and I just think it fuels such fear and panic. I mean, imagine if you were pregnant and someone told you there was a 'risk' of something happening. Scary, right?

Anyway, when we got the screening results back and I had been classed as 'low chance', I don't think it had ever occurred to me that something like that would happen to me. DS just wasn't something I had ever thought about. It's a bit like when you look at other people having horrific car crashes or getting poorly. You look on and think, 'Gosh, that's horrendous,' but mostly you're thinking, 'I couldn't ever imagine that happening to me.' Except here's the thing, shit things happen to people every day: illness, break-ups, losing loved ones. . . the list goes on. And in my forty-three years life on this earth, I've come to realise that none of us is exempt from life not going the way we had planned it, despite my naively thinking that I was untouchable.

And that's the way I saw Oscar and the bombshell of his diagnosis for some time. I'd found myself on a different path to the one I had imagined for myself. I thought my life had taken a dreadful turn for the worse.

When I heard the words, 'I'm so sorry, we suspect your baby has Down syndrome,' I imagined a life sentence. I thought we'd always be sad and that the way others viewed us would be with pity. I spent a lot of time wondering, 'Why us? Why Oscar? Why not anyone else?' Until it dawned on me that there was no rhyme or reason for anything that gets decided for us, so actually. . . why not?

I think a lot of those negative thoughts in the beginning weren't helped by the way Oscar's paediatrician that night had delivered the news. There's no denying I had a fixed view of the way I saw DS myself, which is probably part and parcel of the way that so many of us see DS and what it would mean for us. I saw sadness, no respite and a lot of dribble. And whilst I wasn't expecting a Rockettes-style kickline to announce her suspicions, I often wonder why she didn't at least start with, 'Congratulations'. I'd just had a baby, after all. Wasn't that worth something? In fact, there were no congrats, no mention of the fact that he was beautiful, just an apology. Which indicated to me that she thought this news, for her, would have been the worst imaginable. And, as an impressionable, petrified, first-time mother, lying in a hospital bed, wondering WTF had just happened, that doctor's opinion really mattered to me. I therefore often ponder, would it have been better, after she'd congratulated us and commented on our gorgeous bundle, for her to say something along the lines of, 'Now, the news I'm about to tell you will be unexpected, but please don't panic at this stage. We suspect that Oscar may have Down syndrome.' There really hadn't been any need for the apology.

I guess everyone's different. And whilst DS might be the worst news for some, others may see it as a gift or blessing.

How did she know I didn't feel that way? Who was she to put her unconscious bias on me? (Unconscious bias – counsellor chat!)

Anyway, I digress. The beginning for me was hard. I say 'me' because, from the very start, Chris has been very pragmatic about it all. Oscar's diagnosis isn't something we can change, so the way he's viewed it is to just get on with it. I've often wondered over the past nine years if he might crack, if at any point he might feel hard done by (because I'm going to be honest, when I've been chasing Oscar through our village because I've stupidly given him the benefit of the doubt, left too much space between us and ended up giving it my best Usain Bolt after him, I'm not gonna lie, I've felt hard done by!). But Chris? Never. Not for a minute has he ever resented that our lives with Oscar, on occasion, have been just that little bit harder than if Oscar didn't have that extra chromosome. Not once. And, honestly, I love him a bucketload more for that.

So, those early few weeks and months were tough. I had had this idealistic view of what my new little family was supposed to look like. Only now, I had a disabled son. And now we were 'carers'. I described it as a grief of sorts, which I'm conscious might be an insult to those who have lost a child, but it honestly did feel like someone had ripped my heart out in those first few weeks. I was grieving for the baby I thought I'd have, and it hurt.

For a long time, I resented others who had their 'typical' babies. Every time someone fell pregnant and subsequently had a baby, I found myself wishing that their baby would have DS too, so someone else would understand how I felt. With that, though, came guilt. I sobbed (again to my mum) because I'd find myself thinking these awful things and felt bad that my thoughts could contain such poison.

I remember joining new baby and toddler groups, feeling like it was the right thing to do for me as a new mum and for Oscar's development, only to be faced with huge anxiety about having to introduce myself and explain Oscar's diagnosis. When he was little, I was so conscious of the stares and the apologetic looks. Then there were the people that would avoid all eye contact for fear of what to say or how to react. 'It must be so incredibly hard,' some would say, tilting their heads to one side. All the while I'd be looking at their seemingly perfect baby and their perfect lives and I'd feel jealous.

Things got easier, of course. I realised after a short while that despite it not being the route we'd planned, a mother's love had taken over. In the beginning, Oscar had lots of appointments – mainly medical, to check his heart, his thyroid, his lungs, his hearing, his sight. He had appointments with his consultant paediatrician, his physiotherapist, his occupational therapist and speech therapist. It felt never-ending. But it was around nine months into his little life that we were told the holes in his heart had grown bigger and that he'd need heart surgery. Within a few weeks, we found ourselves at the Royal Brompton Hospital, London, signing the papers for our baby son to have life-saving surgery. That, for me, was the turning point. The moment that I realised that the DS now paled into insignificance. DS was nothing when the thought of losing him was too much even to begin to imagine.

I always talk about Oscar's surgery being huge for me. It was the point when I knew that I loved this baby with my whole heart.

Before I go on, just to fill in a few more gaps. Sixteen-and-a-half months after Oscar, we had another baby, a boy, who we named Alfie. And then, twenty months after that, we had a baby girl, who we called Flo (Florence). In hindsight, I'm almost certain I had Alfie so soon to make up for failings I'd felt the first time round. I had wanted to give Chris the 'perfect' child. I'd wanted our families to feel the euphoria they should have done when I gave birth to Oscar, instead of feeling helpless, and like there was nothing they could do to fix things. I think I thought I wouldn't feel so sad about Oscar's diagnosis if I had a 'typical' baby. Except, when I had Alfie, all I felt was guilty that I'd had him so fast and now my attention was to be shared between my two sons. By the time I had Flo, though, I'd given myself a break. Flo was a much-wanted baby girl, who completed our family, and, once I'd given birth to her, I felt truly genuine happiness, despite us now having three children all in nappies!!!!

And do you know what? Since having three very different children, I've learnt that all children come with their challenges. Diagnosis or not, being a parent to any child is hard. Sure, with the other two there mightn't be flagged 'needs', but there are still worries.

In a lot of ways, Oscar is a much simpler, easier child than the other two. At nine years old, as clichéd as it sounds – and I hate a cliché when it comes to DS as sometimes people assume once they've met one person with DS, they've met them all – he's so happy and content for the most part. Once you've gained his trust, he will love you so completely. With Alfie and Flo there are mood swings; there are manipulative behaviours; they don't always tell the truth. With Oscar, you get what you see: a boy who lives his best life; a boy who finds joy in the unexpected.

In fact, I'm sure we could all do with being a bit more like Oscar. When he feels the music, he dances and sings. When he's in the back of the car, he asks for the window down and he'll sit with his head out of the car and enjoy the feeling of the breeze on his face, where others might close it because it's got too chilly. He has no inhibitions. He'll be the first to walk into a room at a party or approach another child at the park. There is never any agenda with him. He expects others to take him as he is.

We went through some tricky patches with Oz – the biting phase, which lasted a good eighteen months from the age of around two to three-and-a-half, was one of my worst. I became so fearful of taking him to soft play or letting him go on a bouncy castle at another kid's party because we realised that he needed sensory feedback whenever he was playing physically and a bite was his way of getting that. He also bit very intentionally if another child had a toy he wanted. I was, and I suppose only in the last couple of years have I been less of one, a 'helicopter parent'. You know the types, who tend to hover over their kids and become overly involved in their lives. Most 'helicopter parents' do so to pay close attention to their kid's activities and schoolwork, not only to protect them from pain and disappointment, but to help them succeed. I, however, was a 'helicopter parent' to mitigate the risk of Oscar taking a huge chunk out of another kid's arm and me having to deal with that kid's parent, becoming Mother of the Year in their quest to make me feel bad. You probably have no idea how horrified other parents look when your kid takes a chunk out of theirs. Way to make you feel bad or what!!! Thankfully, Oscar grew out of that and, even to this day, when he's on a trampoline or having a game of rough and tumble with Chris, he'll spend the entire time biting his own finger, as he's learnt that's a great way for him to get that sensory feedback and not get in trouble for biting someone. He's a clever sausage.

This book covers where I left off at the end of *For the Love of Oscar*, when Oscar, aged four, had just started school, and brings us up to today, with Oscar aged nine. It's an opportunity to look back and recognise how far he's come, but also to acknowledge some of the challenges along the way. Still, to this day, when he achieves the next milestone, it feels even more special because we know just how much work he's put in to achieve it. We still find magic in this every single time.

Blog Comments

'Grace is the youngest of 4. She does take up our attention quite a lot, but she's 5 so some of that is just being young. But what we didn't realise, was just how much we would all gain! The compassion, tolerance of people who are 'different', seeking justice for those who can't for themselves. Realising how much DS is secondary to who Grace is. It's amazing to watch all my children with her.'

Linda Castle

'Alex (DS) is 25. He has 2 sisters one 27 who he loves with a passion and one 21 who he blames for everything. . . the rain, the traffic. . . He misses them both now they are away living their own lives. They are both very protective of him though. If their friends comment negatively, they cease to be considered friends. I think they would both say they are more rounded people due to having him in their lives.'

Dee Owen-Paxton

'My two are very typical siblings: they look out for each other, get annoyed with each other, play nicely, fight, argue over TV programmes. . . Audrey (DS) is 8 and Rex (neurotypical) is almost 6. I've seen them both stick up for each other at tricky times so I'm confident they'll be a support to each other. At the park some boys were being mean to Rex and Audrey shouted, "STOP BEING MEAN TO MY BROTHER!" – sometimes she has no fear. Another time a kid was trying to pull Audrey's glasses off her face and Rex blocked them, he was only about 2 at the time.'

@vickywooandaudreyboo

2

School Run

I used to think those 'where does the time go?' comments from parents whose kids were starting school were a little annoying, if anything. But now I find myself, one of those parents, literally wondering the very same thing. It doesn't seem five minutes ago that I was sitting in this chair, looking up at Chris behind the camera, smiling on the outside, but my eyes telling a different story. When I look back now, I see a girl needing to be told everything was going to be okay, a girl who needed someone to reassure her that having this teeny, tiny dot of a baby, whom she'd been told just a few hours before was almost certain to have Down syndrome, meant that it wasn't the end of the world, and that the future was a bright one for all of them.

My biggest boy starts school tomorrow. As you can imagine, I'm feeling a mixed bag of emotions right now. At the forefront of my mind this evening is, although I know in my heart of hearts we've made the right decision, there's a little, niggling doubt, wondering if we've done right by him. Will the school we've chosen be too much for him? Will he fit in? Will he struggle there? Will he be understood? Will he understand?

One of the things I find hardest to come to terms with at times is the fact that Oscar can't really articulate to me how he's feeling. Sure, if he's upset or unwell, I know him well enough to know the signs. But if he's unhappy in school, he won't be able to tell me just yet. He can't tell me if someone's been nasty to him or if he's had a bad day and, equally, and just as sad for me, he won't be able to tell me if he's loved his new school and all about any new friends he might have made.

I guess time will tell. I trust the school. They have given me nothing but hope and faith that they have his best interests at heart. And, despite not being able to actually tell me, I have to remember we have done what we thought was best for Oscar at the time.

By the same token, when I think about the diagnosis of Down syndrome we got after he was born and what we thought it meant for him, I never, for one moment, dreamt he'd be the little boy he's become today.

* * * *

Tuesday 6 September 2016 – Oscar's first day in reception class at our local village infant school. We had toyed with sending him to other schools in the area, but our heart had been set on sending him to our local school as we felt it would be lovely for Oscar to be known in our community and we desperately wanted Oscar to have the opportunity to be with his little brother and sister once they started school, even for a short time. We'd also thought about sending him to a specialist school, but, having looked around a couple, at that stage, we'd decided that they weren't for him. When we'd looked at other mainstream schools, despite their saying all the right things on their websites, noting how inclusive and accepting they were of all children, some couldn't have made it more obvious that they didn't want a child like Oscar there. I remember emailing the headteacher of our local school when Oscar was just a few months old, asking if they'd be happy to take him, desperate for him to be like any other child back then. The fact that I emailed her when he was so tiny screamed of that desperation. She'd said yes, and I have since learnt that they'd had a little girl with DS there previously.

There'd been meetings set up before Oscar started. Professionals like his physio, speech therapist, occupational therapist and educational psychologist had got involved. We hadn't quite managed to get his EHCP (Educational Health and Care Plan) in place before he started as I was still fighting for speech and language provision, but we did know that he had been awarded full-time one-on-one support (32.5 hours a week), who would be with him the entire time he was at school, e.g. in the classroom and to cover breaks and lunchtimes.

Like any first-time mum, I'd been apprehensive in the run-up to Oscar starting school. Being a July baby, he was just four. He was preverbal, with only a handful of Makaton signs (and even these were Oscar's own versions), and he was still in nappies, nowhere near ready to use the toilet independently. I'd been worried because, even though the school had said they were happy to take him and had done everything they could to provide for his personal-care needs, I appreciated how different it would be for them having a child like Oz there.

When Oscar was tiny, we were advised to start using Makaton with him. Makaton is a language programme using signs and symbols to aid communication. Naively, it was the first time I'd ever heard of it and, to be honest,

I questioned whether it was necessary. I think, in the beginning, I'd been in denial that Oscar would need additional help. But Makaton is put in place to support a child's speech – words are still spoken in addition to the signing – so speeds up and develops language-learning for children with speech delay.

Today, over 100,000 children and adults use Makaton symbols and signs, either as their main method of communication or to support speech. In addition to children and adults with communication and learning difficulties and the communities around them – teachers, health professionals, friends and public service bodies – Makaton is increasingly used by the general public to aid communication.

That first year, Oscar was assigned two teaching assistants, which I had agreed was a good idea. One would cover the morning and one the afternoon. I'd loved the morning one, who ended up being assigned to Oz off and on for the next four years. She had been a teacher previously, was so proactive in her approach to learning Makaton (something the school weren't trained in but subsequently tried to introduce) and I had faith in her from the start that she had Oscar's best interests and his progression at the forefront of everything she did.

After his first day, the report-back was that he had done brilliantly. Although he looked a little unsure, there had been no tears when he went in. He just gave us a hug goodbye and off he went. I don't think he even looked back, completely unfazed by the whole thing. He explored the classroom for the first ten minutes, then settled down, playing in the home corner, interacting with his new classmates. He got a little teary in the last five minutes of the session but I'm guessing he was feeling tired after all the excitement of the morning. All in all, though, a big success and a huge relief on my part. I'd been relieved that he'd settled so well, but also that I hadn't completely lost it. No one tells you how big a deal seeing your first-born head off to school is and how emotional you'll find yourself. I suppose it's the end of an era and you're handing your pride and joy into the hands of someone else for most of the week. Add in the fact that Oscar couldn't yet tell me how he'd got on because he hadn't yet got the speech to let me know and that was a lot to deal with emotionally.

By the end of the first week, I hoped I wasn't speaking too soon, but we were all happy. From the expression on his face when he ran out to greet me after he'd finished for the day, he seemed so at home. Although, to start with, he was doing only a few hours a day at a time, I think the change and the new routine hit him that first Friday evening as he was asleep on the sofa by 6 p.m.

In the mornings, he managed the ten-minute walk to school with no problems. I had been dubious initially, worrying about him running off, especially because it was a busy time of day with all the extra school traffic on both the roads and the pavements. But he'd walk alongside me and it was interesting to see that when he saw other children holding their mummies' hands, he'd wanted to hold mine, something he would never normally have instigated.

On that Friday morning of the first week, however, when he stepped out of the front door, he signed that he wanted to get in the car and got a little tearful when I said we had to walk. Thankfully, he got a ride on the buggy-board of the buggy I was pushing Alfie and Flo in, and he'd perked up by the time we got to school. As time went on and Oscar got more confident with where he was going each morning, the walk to school became problematical.

To bystanders, things may have looked calm and collected. Oscar would walk just a short distance in front of me as I'd be pushing the double buggy with Alfie and Flo in, and some days, as his mother, I'd totally got everything under control.

Oscar's a creature of habit. He knew to stop at the roads we had to cross. I would always give him a vocal cue – 'Oscar, STOP!' (usually shrieked at the top of my voice, just in case) and he would do so well with stopping, before we checked for traffic. He liked to climb on some of the small walls outside a couple of the shops on the village high street and he'd gesture to me to hold his hand to help him balance. He would occasionally take a little detour into our local branch of the Co-op and decide it was time to grab a basketful of essentials, but was usually compliant when I told him that we didn't need any shopping that morning.

On other mornings, he may have been found wandering up to the entrance of the fruit and veg shop to say hi, but then they'd often give him a free banana, so why wouldn't he do that. . . he's not stupid, right?

The walk home was a different story and fast becoming an Olympic sprint. It started with a downhill pursuit – did I mention the school is on a hill? – involving Oscar darting off, closely followed by me, and my double buggy, jogging after him. I say jogging as I didn't want to alert the oncoming fellow parents on their way to pick up their kids that I/we were completely out of control and that this kid may have outsmarted me. I would try to remain calm as I negotiated my way around them all: small children, dogs on leads, scooters and the occasional, unassuming elderly man or woman, who really didn't need to be run over by me. Oscar, it seemed, had mastered the art of weaving in and out of all these people, all the while occasionally looking behind, checking that I was keeping up. He was grinning from ear to ear and clearly finding it hilarious that mummy was running (jogging obviously sped up) in hot pursuit. My ever-increasing anxiety over the school run was getting worse. It seemed the more confident he got, the more distance there would be between us and the less safe it felt. Despite imploring him repeatedly to hold the buggy, he simply wouldn't. The turning point for me was when we had a near miss.

On the way to school on this morning, along a narrow pavement, Oscar had got ahead of me and the buggy and ducked in front of another parent with her two children. To this day, he still has this thing that he hates walking behind people. If there's someone walking ahead of us, he has to get in front of them, which is fine when it's just one other person, but on a crowded school run? Nightmare! The double buggy was heavy and hard to handle with Alfie and Flo in it. I'd realised that there was no way I'd be able to get to him as I'd have to navigate the buggy off the pavement and into oncoming traffic, so I held my breath, just hoping he'd stop. But before I knew it, he'd darted across the road at the traffic lights. . . and they weren't on red.

Mercifully, although it was busy, there were no cars on the road at the time, but my heart was pounding in my chest. He had never done that before and I'm not sure what it was that made him decide to cross the road – we didn't need to – but that was the final straw and the moment when I decided, in the interest of his personal safety, that I'd have to put him on a rein, for a while at least, until he understood the dangers. We had done this when he was younger, but the trouble was that he was so physically able and had grown so much in confidence over the last few months that I was reluctant to take this step. Unfortunately, though, I couldn't be sure that he understood the consequences of his actions, and the terrible accident that could so easily have happened that morning. I also realised that my desire to allow him to be as 'normal' as possible and walk like the other children had endangered his life. That was unforgivable on my part. So, after giving my ego a stern talking to, the next day I found his old backpack with a strap attached, packed a packet of Mini Cheddars for the walk home, and he was as good as gold. Lesson well and truly learnt.

The following morning, he even went and got his school uniform and shoes to change into, without me mentioning school and over the weekend, when we drove past the school, he pointed and shouted, 'Mum, Mum, Mum, Yeeeeeeeeeah!'

For the record, the only other places he lets out a cheer when we drive past or arrive at are the park, Nanny and Grumps' house and an ice cream van. So, I think I can say with confidence that school had got a big thumbs up.

That first term was like a rollercoaster: so many highs and lows along the way. The school had started a communication diary in which the teaching assistants, teachers and I could write down and share information on how a day had gone or what sort of weekend or night Oscar had had. This was something that I knew would be extremely helpful to all of us. I realised, though, that I'd be holding my breath every day when he came out, anxious to hear how he'd got on, wanting so badly for him to fit in alongside the other children.

Walking in to school one morning, I heard a little voice behind us call out, 'Oscar. . . Hi, Oscar. Mummy, look, it's Oscar.'

We turned round to say hello and a little girl, who happened to be in Oscar's class, came running up behind him to give him a big hug. Clearly chuffed with his new admirer, Oscar continued to hug the little girl as they walked along – no mean feat, I might add – as they made their way to the school gate.

'Oscar's flavour of the month at the moment,' the little girl's mummy told me.

'Oh, really?' I said. 'That's so lovely.'

'Yes, she tells me Oscar always gives lovely hugs. . . and he's the best dancer.'

Little interactions like this one meant so much, and five years on, they still do. One of my biggest fears when Oscar started mainstream school was that he wouldn't have any friends. So little moments like this one were precious.

A few weeks in Oscar caught a cold. It was inevitable as he was often so susceptible to colds and chest infections when he was younger and, with the change in the weather and the setting, it was a given. His paediatrician had put him on Azithromycin, a low-dose antibiotic that he and a lot of children who happen to have DS take during the winter months to keep chest infections at bay. It helped during these early years.

During this same week, I had had a meeting with Oscar's 'new' educational psychologist ('new' as this was his third in only eighteen months), along with his two class teachers. His teacher opened the meeting with, 'If only all the children were as good with routine as Oscar is. . . he's doing brilliantly.' I nearly fell off my chair. Apparently, they had some sort of rain stick that they shook to signify certain instructions and he'd really responded to it. When it was time for the children to line up, he would whizz straight over to do so. When it was time to get his fruit at snack time, he was on it and cleaned up beautifully afterwards, putting his Tupperware back in the box. That took me back a little, as, for anyone who knows Oscar well, 'conforming' and 'doing what he's told' isn't always something you'd necessarily associate with him, so this made me super-proud and happy to hear.

They noted, though, that 'carpet time' was harder for Oscar. He found it really challenging to sit for any extended amount of time, but they'd developed some strategies that meant he was building up the time he'd sit still for. Some days were obviously better than others, but they'd been working on increasing that time little by little.

By the sounds of things, Oscar had been a little reluctant to do some of the one-on-one tasks outside of the classroom. The school and I had had a discussion before he started about the fact that, although we didn't want him to spend hours out of the class, there would be times he wouldn't be able to keep up with what the rest of the class were doing, and that time would be better spent doing a table activity outside the classroom. His morning teaching assistant had set up an area under the stairs, which, although it sounds very much like Harry Potter's childhood, was a lovely workspace for him to go and have some quiet time. She'd decorated it with Mr Tumble picture cards, which he loved, and it meant so much to us at the time that she'd gone to so much effort. However, his reluctance to go out there sometimes probably had more to do with the appeal of a busy classroom, which must have appeared a lot more exciting than having to sit down quietly to do his matching or sequences. All in all, though, five weeks in and they said he appeared to have settled well, seemed happy and was apparently a big hit with the Year One girls. That's my boy!

And on his first class trip, to watch *The Tortoise and the Hare* at our local theatre, aside from initially being a little apprehensive going in, the report-back was that he had sat beautifully for the entire duration of the show.

At the end of Oscar's first half-term at infant school, with an hour to go before I picked him up, just when I thought everything was going smoothly, Oscar got himself into a spot of trouble. Having been involved in no biting incidents all term, Oscar had bitten one of the little girls in his class. At breaktime, he'd gone into the playhouse in the playground. A group of girls had followed him in and, we were told, they had been trying to hug Oscar. Guessing he'd felt trapped and, because he didn't have the verbal communication to tell them to stop, he took a bite out of one of his admirers. Luckily, it didn't break the skin and the little girl was fine, but I felt really deflated. He'd done so well up until this point. Yet, with just a few minutes to go before the end of school, Jaws was back.

Aside from this little blip, Chris and I were immensely proud of our little man. Not only did he appear to be loving school, but the teachers had also said he'd done so well. The morning teaching assistant also said that if something hadn't worked, she had adapted things to suit Oscar, but had also been mindful to keep him on task. When we'd arrive at school in the mornings, he would be greeted by fellow students shouting, 'Hi, Oscar', mostly from different year groups and classes. We'd noticed at home that he was playing with toys more. His focus and attention, although still a work in progress, seemed to be improving and he was even bringing books to us to read to him. This was unheard of previously; he'd never been a 'let's sit down quietly and read' type of kid. I'd felt disheartened that afternoon when we had our setback, but when I looked at the big picture and thought about how many things he had achieved over the past few months and how far he'd come, I couldn't help but smile.

Blog Comments

'Seb is in Year 9 at mainstream secondary. For me, it's about keeping an open mind and taking each day at a time. It's working well now – but not without a few challenges. I personally feel like no route is completely perfect. There are things Seb misses out on at mainstream, but he gains things he wouldn't get at special school. It was without doubt the most anxiety-inducing part of our journey so far choosing which school but thankfully, so far, it's working out.'

Carly White

'My mainstream school would not be the place it is without our pupils with DS. We are lost when they are off school for illness etc. They bring so much joy, compassion, fun and learning to our community. They are an equal, unique and a very important part of our school family.'

Headteacher of a mainstream junior school

'I work across six mainstream schools as their speech therapist. The schools employ me directly and have a superb executive SENCO who used to be head at a special school, and we are employing ex-special schoolteachers as SENCOs to get the expertise into our schools. We now have non-verbal autistic children coming to us and, whilst a challenge for all, it is a challenge that, with the correct support, teachers are rising to. We are creating

---

environments where I wish my daughter had gone to mainstream. She has moved from mainstream to special after doing her GCSEs. I can safely say she has made no academic progress; they lump her in with all other needs and there are no specialist DS methods employed. I am also friends with a lovely special schoolteacher with five girls in her class of 8 with DS. She has no idea of any of the specialist interventions for children with DS and I find this is a problem, as they aren't learning to read, aren't being encouraged to learn, and are working on "life skills" which have their place, but the school years are for developing learning skills as well.'

Anon

'Finlay attended 2 provisions during his preschool year – one mainstream and one specialist. I hoped it would help me to decide but he fitted in well. We decided on mainstream in the end with our minds always open to switching to specialist when the time was right. I never expected that he would still be there to the end of year 6 and was convinced that he would go to a specialist school for secondary education. Yet here we are now, one term of year 7 completed in a mainstream secondary school. It's not all been plain sailing but communication with the SENCo and class teachers is key. I have days when I think of pulling him out and moving to a specialist school, but my biggest problem is that he doesn't fit in any of the local specials. He's been in mainstream for 7 years. He knows how to navigate there. He is capable of learning there and it's vital for him to have peers who can be role models. My friends whose kids go to special schools frequently comment that their children are not pushed academically. Finlay has the capability to achieve academically, and I don't want to take that away.'

Helen McCann

'Special education isn't a building. I'll do a happy dance on the day we stop with the notion of "mainstream" schools and think more inclusively. This is very nuanced for our community. Many of our parents haven't had choice for their children, often their kids are discriminated against even in the first school conversations "your child doesn't fit", "we don't fit your child", "the gap will increase", "we can't meet their needs". As it stands, the education system certainly lets down so many pupils. We must be more aspirational for more pupils and how do we expect to raise capable and aspirational carers (doctors, nurses etc.) if they don't get to intermix with a greater range of ppl with AN (additional needs) as they both grow and develop?! How do they nurture their caring tendencies?!'

Lynne Murray

3

Be Kind

'The potential for greatness lives within each of us'
Wilma Rudolph

I was out shopping with Flo – the boys were at preschool and school – when I spotted a little boy with Down syndrome. Looking at him, I guessed he was around ten years old and, like some sort of crazy stalker, I stood and watched as he and his mum interacted with one another. I'd joined the ridiculously long queue in Zara to pay, so I had plenty of time to people-watch and there, almost directly in front of me, was this boy. I watched as his mum picked out outfits for him and he stood with her obviously saying yes or no to what she was picking out. He got involved himself, picking up a few outfits that he liked. I was there for about ten minutes (yep, doing brilliantly with the old queue control, Zara!) and for the whole duration, I didn't at any point feel like his mum was struggling to keep an eye on him. He didn't once wander off or make a dash for it out of the front door. They were both relaxed; he chatted to her and, from the point of view of an outsider looking in, he couldn't have been better behaved if he'd tried.

Standing in a busy shopping centre with Oscar by my side, perusing the rails of Zara, felt like a million miles off for us back then. I couldn't begin to imagine not having to keep an eye on Oscar in that situation, not even for a second. So, standing in that queue, I felt some hope, that one day, Oz and I would have that with one another. I'd thought about going over and saying all this to the boy's mum, but I decided to leave them to it. (I didn't have Oz with me and I always find it a bit odd striking up a conversation with another parent of a child with DS. It's like, 'Hey, I've got one of those at home too!' I mean, what *do* you say in those situations?) Anyway, I vowed that day that the next time I was reminding Oscar, for the thirty-sixth time that year, to walk in a straight line to school and not to run off into our local Co-op and complete a circuit of the entire shop, just for laughs, that I'd remember that boy and how much he made me smile.

In the nine years I've been a parent to three very different children, I've learnt that friendships aren't always a given. Flo, my youngest, is very social. At six years old, with blonde hair and blue eyes, she has always managed to charm the adults around her and hold her own in a friendship group, despite being one of the youngest in her year. Alfie, aged eight, on the other hand, finds it harder. He has friends, but a select few, and it's only in the last year or so that he'd instigate conversation or play in the park with another child, whilst Flo would approach anyone who'd listen from day dot. Oscar is a sociable little boy, who'll happily start joining in a kick-about in the park, without showing signs of any inhibitions whatsoever. In fact, just recently, when Alfie had wanted to join in a game of football at the park, with a bunch of children he didn't know, he'd asked me to go and get Oscar, who was happily playing in the playground, to get him to approach them and join in, so he could too. But whilst with typical kids, as a parent, you have faith that they'll navigate friendships and find their way, with a child who has additional needs, there's always that fear that they won't have friends, particularly for someone like Oscar, who still had very few words.

Oscar's approach to friendships wasn't conventional. I'll never forget the time a mum of one of the little girls in Oscar's school came up to me in the playground and said, 'My daughter loves Oscar and says he's so funny.'

Knowing Oscar as I did, I'd been reluctant to ask her to define the word 'funny', but obviously being too inquisitive not to ask, I said, 'Oh really, why does she think he's funny?' To which she replied, 'Because she says he likes to sit on her,'!!!

I once read about three five-year-old little girls, who were standing in a circle having a chat. One of the children had Down syndrome and one of the girls was explaining to the other why their friend was different from them both. I'd read that she'd said, 'She doesn't understand things because her brain doesn't work properly.'

I'll leave you to ponder that and come back to it in a minute.

Shortly after Oscar started school, he, Alfie and Flo were playing at a children's playground. Oscar *loves* older kids. He always has done and will often stand and watch them on their skateboards or climbing on all the high play equipment in awe. On this occasion, when Oscar spotted a little girl he thought looked nice, he ran over to the swing next to her, smiling as he went and, as soon as he sat down, she looked at him and ran off looking scared. Although I felt a pang in my heart that I probably would have done if any of my kids had been blatantly rebuffed like that, Oscar, seemingly unfazed, carried on playing, and I continued shadowing him around the playground. But what had happened next really hit a raw nerve. There was a tunnel that the kids could crawl through and on top of the tunnel there was a big mound of earth that a few of the children were climbing up on top of and looking out across the park. There was a boy standing on top of the mound, I'd say around nine or ten years old and, as Oscar started to climb up, I had a feeling Oscar wanted to 'talk' to the boy. I watched, smiling, as Oscar stood next to the boy and gently placed his hand on his shoulder. Peering round to look up at his face, he said, 'Hiya.' It was the sweetest moment, and anyone who has a child who struggles with verbal communication will understand the poignancy of this, I'm sure.

The older boy's mother was sitting on a bench no further than a few feet away. I knew it was his mum as they'd spoken together previously and, just a few seconds earlier, we'd made eye contact before she'd turned back to look at the boys.

As Oscar said, 'Hiya,' I had expected this boy, being that bit older, to turn around and say hello back. Only he didn't. He shifted nervously, looked away from Oscar and froze, until Oscar took his hand off his shoulder.

'Are you saying hi, Oscar?' I asked him. 'Yeah,' he shouted back to me. Thinking that if I interrupted, the boy might feel a bit more comfortable to say hello. Or, failing that, his mother, sitting just a short distance away, would step in and say to her son, 'Say hi to the little boy.'

Only he didn't. And neither did she. And both, as I looked over at her, seemed as disgusted as each other by the interaction. I didn't need to say any more and quickly distracted Oscar by saying, 'Let's go and play in the sand,' but, in much the same way as I was by the girl on the swing's reaction to Oscar, I felt hurt for him.

And the thing is, I did get that Oscar could sometimes be a bit full on. If they'd been watching him in the playground, which I imagine they must have been doing leading up to their interactions, he wasn't holding back. When he's having fun, even still today, he'll charge from one piece of apparatus to the next. If he wants to say hi to someone, he will, whereas I guess typically developing kids might be just that little more reserved. As an aside, I absolutely love this about him and wish I had half his energy and 'I don't give two hoots' attitude. And I really got that kids might find this too much and, although it made me sad for Oscar, I understood why the girl on the swing ran away and why the boy on top of the mound didn't acknowledge Oz. They were kids after all.

But what I *didn't* get, not for one single second, is why the mother didn't step in and encourage her son to say hello, why she thought it was okay at his age, an age when, surely, he should know better than to ignore someone when they're talking to him, not to step in and say something? But then I remembered her facial expression and realised she'd not known how to deal with Oscar either.

I then recalled the conversation between the five-year-olds that I'd read about and realised that 'her brain doesn't work properly' weren't words that would have come from the young girl; they could only have come from an adult, whom I assume was one of her parents, which then made me ponder, 'Is there any hope for kids if their parents' attitudes are so narrow-minded?'

So, here's the thing: if you're a parent of a child, whatever their age, can we teach them to be kind, please? Can we teach them that 'different' is okay and that being around 'difference' is nothing to be feared? Can we teach them about patience and understanding too, please? And when we're explaining about a child they may know from school, or the park, or who they've seen in the street or have just met, can we be mindful of our choice of words – mindful of our own attitudes, I guess. For I'm certain that if any of us is reluctant to say hello or we feel awkward ourselves, our attitude will be shared by our kids.

I wonder if – before I had Oscar – I might not have known what to say and how to be? Who knows? But I vowed that if there was one thing that I was going to try to be my absolute best at, it was to teach all three of my kids that kindness and understanding really do go a long, long way.

During the half-term break, with the help of my mum, who was never too far away at this stage of my life, I organised some day trips. On one occasion, we'd spent the day at Wisley Gardens as they'd had an *In the Night Garden* tent. First, the children were read an interactive story. They then had a little dance and music class with instruments to play; to finish off, they did a yoga session. It was just the sweetest thing! There was also an *In the Night Garden* trail to find our favourite characters which we could have done too, but most of our time was spent looking at the tractors on display, and in the area for the kids to play on diggers, which had a whole heap of muddy earth to move in wheelbarrows. The kids *loved* it!

Considering that, before I'd left the house that day, I was having mild palpitations at the thought of being able to control the children and not lose any of them amongst the hordes of other people enjoying their half terms, we did well. Oh, and ironically after the park trip a couple of days beforehand, this time, when Oscar approached a little boy to say, 'Hello', the boy said, 'Hello,' straight back. As we walked away, I heard him say to his mum, 'That's my new friend, Mummy,' which, both for me and my faith in humanity, couldn't have been more perfectly timed.

Just before Oscar's first term ended, he took part in his first ever nativity play at school. If I'm completely honest, I wasn't holding out much hope that it'd be a success. Over the course of the years, although he was a confident little boy in many ways, as he'd grown older and, I suppose, a bit more 'aware', when we'd asked him to try anything new, it would take him some time to adjust. His first reaction was to run or shy away.

The performance was taking place in our local village church, just across from the school, so I'd wondered initially if he'd even enter the building, let alone walk in with a big, broad grin plastered across his face. He'd never been a fan of big crowds, but the fact that the church was full of parents and grandparents didn't seem to faze him at all. After many disastrous attempts at getting him into various Halloween fancy-dress costumes, mainly for my amusement and photo opportunities, he would normally flatly refuse to wear any outfit. But for the nativity play he wore his shepherd costume without any fuss at all – although he did refuse to wear his headdress. The performance was forty-five minutes in total. Forty-five minutes would be a long time for any four-year-old to sit still for, but for Oscar, at this stage, forty-five minutes must have felt like an eternity, and was super-difficult for him.

As the nativity went on, depending on which characters they were, the children had to go up and down the aisles acting out the story – first Mary, Joseph and the donkey, next the stars, then the angels, followed by the villagers and, finally, it was the turn of the shepherds. As I said, I wasn't holding my breath that Oz would join in or do any of the actions but then suddenly, there he was, without his morning teaching assistant who obviously believed he could do his bit without her help, walking down the aisle, copying his peers as he went. He spotted me almost straight away and I thought that might be the point when he decided that he'd had enough, but no, he carried on with the actions. Then, when it was time to go back to his seat, he turned around to me, gave me a big wave and shouted, 'Bye,' as if it was no big deal at all.

He took part in two performances that day. The first at 9.30 a.m. and the second later that evening at 5.30 p.m. I thought he'd be past it by then, to be honest, but I watched as he smiled his way through the second performance too. For me, watching Oscar up there was a pinnacle moment, a memory that I will cherish forever. My heart was bursting with pride and, as he walked back to his seat to sit with his class and turned to me and waved, tears streamed down my face. Never, in those moments after receiving his diagnosis, did I imagine my heart would feel this happy. But it did, more than ever before.

Blog Comments

'Caleb is in mainstream in Year 10 and has a variety of friends, both with special needs and without. We've had to help him to make the effort at times over the years and I'm aware lots of work was put in by schools when he was younger. He's excellent with names and although he's a little slower in picking up social cues he gets there.'

Marianne Holt

'Cara's in Year 1 in MS [mainstream] school, and she has a couple of best friends, but she also works hard to interact with the other children in her class. One of the things that school has done which is good, is focused on helping Cara to ask others to play with her and giving her the language for those social interactions. I think that's been great for her.'

Meryn Brown

'We don't have the option of a SEN school, but Levi is doing great in mainstream. He is in 5th grade and his friendships have stayed strong. The other kids look out for him and help him when he is struggling or needs guidance. It is amazing to watch them accommodate him all on their own without being told.'

Bobbi Rees Olivett

4

Two bananas, a box of raisins, three packets of Fruit Stars, a packet of Pom-Bears, a packet of Quavers, six Oreo Thins, two sausages and a jelly

'I'm not an early bird or a night owl. I'm some form of permanently exhausted pigeon'
Unknown

I often say, if I was on *Mastermind*, (I mean, obviously highly unlikely, but sometimes these things spring into my head), 'Sleep' would be my specialist subject. Sleep or, more to the point, Oscar's *lack of* sleep, was all-consuming. Just after I'd had Flo, when Oscar had recently turned three, his sleeping patterns took a turn for the worse.

I remember bringing Oscar back from hospital and him being able to self-settle. He'd spent ten days in NICU (Neonatal Intensive Care Unit), had been tube fed with a combination of boob and bottle and when I or the nurses would put him down, he'd doze off, no trouble at all. Lots of people said it was because he was a heart baby. He had two holes in his heart and feeding for him was a lot of effort. By the time he was done, he was exhausted and would drift off. I think also the fact that he was on such a strict routine back then – fed every three hours, winded and put back in his incubator, he just adjusted. When he was discharged from hospital, the 2012 London Olympics were on telly. It was such an odd time. There was the euphoria I'd felt watching the games, mixed with the happiness of having a newborn baby, combined with a deep-rooted sadness that wouldn't leave me, an overwhelming sense that life would now look very different for me and my little family. I recall putting Oscar's Moses basket on the other side of the living room so that he wouldn't get disturbed by the noise of the television. But he was no bother. After his feeds, he'd drift back off to sleep without any fuss.

As he grew a little older, he liked us to rock him to sleep, but Chris and I would joke that after two minutes' worth of 'step touching' (I am an ex-dancer so we had turned to rocking him in our arms in a dance routine), he'd be off. In those days, whilst the rest of my NCT (National Childbirth Trust) group would be exchanging emails at 2 a.m., discussing how their babies had been up for hours, I was getting full, uninterrupted nights of sleep and Oz was only around eight weeks old. The paediatrician, dietician (Oscar had a dietician as he wasn't putting on much weight) and health visitor all told me I should be waking him to try to get some milk into him. But he was so dozy that even when I managed to wake him, he would never take that much.

Apart from the not-putting-on-weight thing, which he managed eventually when he was placed on a fortifier to build him up, he was literally the dream baby. He would sleep from 8 p.m. to 8 a.m. and I remember smugly thinking, 'What's up with everyone stressing about newborn's sleep? I've hit the jackpot.' But, of course, as every smug, annoying mum knows, being that smug backfires every time, as when Oscar hit three and, with my newborn Flo thrown into the mix, his sleep went massively downhill.

I think initially our problem was that he was getting up at 5 a.m. Every single morning. No matter what time we put him down, from a very young age, he's always been up with the lark. And that doesn't bother me, if we've had a good night; only we were finding that it was taking him a couple of hours to go to sleep and then, subsequently, he was waking numerous times in the night, too.

When he was around three years old, he was prescribed melatonin. This was to help him go to sleep, as we were finding we were having to sit with him for ages whilst he fell asleep. I should also point out that this all coincided with his having worked out how to climb out of his cot, so we'd switched him to a bed and he now wouldn't stay put without us lying with him and would be constantly up and down. The melatonin worked in that he fell asleep a lot quicker, but I went on to have years and years of *horrendously* interrupted sleep. You'll be pleased to hear that it has got much better now that Oscar has reached the grand old age of nine. Last year, after another call to his paediatrician, he was prescribed Phenergan. And whilst he still has periods of bad sleep, which I used to think were the result of ear infections but honestly who knows, the Phenergan, when he's fully well, and, by that, I mean ear-infection- and cold-free, has been a real life saver for us. I say us, but I mean me, as Oz seems to be able to survive on very little sleep and Chris, who is the heaviest sleeper in the land, has had a full nine hours sleep a night, just about every night, for the past nine years!!!! Must be nice, hey?

I have always said, and this might sound harsh, I can handle a lot of the challenges that come with having a child with DS – the speech delays, the biting, the long-winded toilet training (no pun intended), but lack of sleep, I swear, has nearly killed me off. They say sleep deprivation is a form of torture and I would wholeheartedly agree.

Anyway, the problem was that around the time Oscar started school, he'd still be waking every morning around 5 a.m., but he would also wake up during the night, anything from a couple of times to six times a night! Yep, sometimes *six* times. Typically, his sleeping usually got worse when he was about to be, or was, poorly, which was obviously understandable and not something I would ever resent him for, but then sometimes he could wake six times for no apparent reason whatsoever.

And usually, I would have just got on with it. When others said to me, 'Gosh I don't know how you do it?' – another thing that gets my back up, but I'll come on to that later – I've shrugged and said, 'I don't really have a choice.' And I've realised that since having kids, you can survive on very little sleep if you need to. But then occasionally, sleep deprivation could send me over the edge. My husband Chris can attest to this, having been on the receiving end.

Something that I truly believe impacted on Oscar's sleep was the bombshell discovery that he had cholesteatoma. Just before he started school, because Oscar's hearing had been repeatedly down and his speech really wasn't coming on, Chris, myself and Oscar's ENT consultant made the decision to fit him with grommets. This is quite a controversial procedure on a child who happens to have DS as their ear canals are significantly smaller than their typically developing peers and they therefore don't always have the best success rate, as the grommets can fall out. We wanted to give it a go, though, as I'd heard for some children with DS, the grommets had worked, and their speech had really taken off afterwards. In retrospect, I'm so grateful we did, as had we not gone for the surgery, the cholesteatoma might never have been found and that could have had a big impact.

In layman's terms, cholesteatoma is an abnormal collection of skin cells deep inside the ear. They're rare, but if left untreated, they can damage the delicate structures inside the ear that are essential for hearing and balance. A cholesteatoma can also lead to ear infections, causing discharge from the ear. The other worry was that bone erosion can cause the infection to spread into the surrounding areas, including the inner ear and brain. If untreated, deafness, brain abscess, meningitis, and, although rare, even death can occur.

In January 2017, just after Oscar started school, he had intensive surgery to remove the cholesteatoma. At this stage it was in only one ear, but his surgeon had described it as a weed, in that if even the smallest part was left, it would keep growing, spread further and do significant damage to his inner ear. After the surgery, I got home at 10.30 p.m. It had been a long day, the surgery having lasted five hours and thirty minutes, a lot longer than we and his ENT team had anticipated. Chris stayed in the hospital with him overnight. Oscar adores Chris and we knew that he would be happy to have Daddy with him if he were to wake in the night.

Thankfully, the operation went well, though. They managed to get the cholesteatoma all out and were happy, but said it was a very difficult, intricate job because of how tiny his ear was. There was obviously also a chance it could grow back which meant he'd need follow-up surgery in nine months to a year to check it hadn't. The way they had gone in was to cut from behind the top of his ear to the bottom and then pulled back the entire ear to see what was going on. It sounded gruesome and for a while his ear stuck out whilst the swelling went down. They had also packed his ear with gauze which he was to have in for the following three weeks, before getting it removed (again under general anaesthetic). And until then, we were warned, he'd only be able to hear out of one ear. The good news, though, was that he had now had a titanium implant inserted as the disease had eroded a lot of the components that make up the ear. The doctors said that once the packing was removed, after a few weeks, his hearing should improve.

Oscar was discharged the following day and we kept him off school. He was still quite emotional and wanted a lot of cuddles, which wasn't really like him at all. He'd had a reasonable night's sleep in the hospital, but it looked like rolling onto his side was causing him pain and he'd always liked to move around a lot in bed. We kept up with the Calpol and Ibuprofen regularly, so during the daytime he seemed comfortable enough. His ear was still very swollen, though, and when Chris and I left him on his own briefly that afternoon, when we walked back into the room, we found him looking very sheepish. On closer inspection we realised he'd managed to pull some of the packing out of his ear, which wasn't ideal as it was still quite gross. We called his surgeon's office to check this wasn't a major issue and they said to put some cotton wool back in his ear with some Vaseline on it and it would be okay.

Oscar received a big card from his class at school. They'd all drawn him a little picture and signed their name. Also, that afternoon there was a knock at the door and his teaching assistant had come round with a card and the latest Mr Tumble magazine. People were so kind.

A few weeks later, under general anaesthetic, Oscar had the packing removed from his ear. They also used it as a chance to see how the ear was healing and to check on the titanium implant. While he was asleep, I asked them to check on the grommet they'd inserted in the other ear, to see if it was still in place. Thankfully the grommet was still there, and all looked great with the ear they'd operated on. He had a hearing test scheduled for a few months later, as it was going to take around that long for the implant to start working properly and for his hearing to hopefully improve. After that, he'd been asked to go back to see his ENT consultant.

Oscar was pretty good that day. You'd have thought that over the years of various surgeries – heart, testes, belly-button hernia, ears – that he'd be a pro and take it all in his stride, but I think it's just made him more suspicious of anyone wearing scrubs or carrying a stethoscope. He's never been a fan of doctors or nurses, so any time an anaesthetist tries to put him under, invariably he loses it. This was okay when he was tiny, because I was able to give him a cuddle and putting the mask over his face was straightforward.

Fast forward to age nine, when he had a routine op to check what was going on in his ears (he's been getting recurring ear infections for some time now) and he lost it. Picture the scene: I'm sat on the bed, legs akimbo – mine, not his – with him sat in between, and me trying to squeeze him in some sort of wrestling manoeuvre. A play therapist was holding his iPad so he could continue watching CBeebies and Oscar was getting *so* stressed. You may notice I say 'I' as in, I'm the one who gets the treat of putting Oz under. Chris is an amazing dad, but he hates watching Oscar go under general anaesthetic. He says he finds it too emotional and gets too upset. And by that he means him!!! So, like a mug, I say I'll do it every time;

and every time, much like when I take Oscar for his six-monthly blood test (Chris hates watching Oscar having his blood taken, too), I am cursing Chris as I sweat from every orifice and am trying, myself, not to cry. I've decided that I could just about hold it together if doctors, nurses and anaesthetists weren't so bloody lovely. Once he's asleep and it's all calm and you can feel yourself on the brink, all you want to do is run out of that room before anyone notices you're teary. . . but they insist on telling you how brilliant you are, how brave and how they'll look after him for you. And then, that's it, game over and the waterworks start. Damn them for being so nice.

This time, Oscar got very cross before he went down to surgery, as stupidly I'd left his lunchbox of food out where he could see it (obviously, before a procedure you can't eat). Well, you'd have thought the world had ended. Major meltdown. He'd made up for it when he woke up though, eating the entire contents of the box – two bananas, a box of raisins, three packets of Fruit Stars, a packet of Pom-Bears, a packet of Quavers and six Oreo Thins (who knew they were so nice?). Oh, and he then had two sausages and a jelly that the hospital provided at tea-time. This boy can eat.

A few months after his first cholesteatoma surgery, it was time to test his hearing again. Two audiologists were present. One sat at a little table, distracting Oscar with toys, while the other operated the sound board. To begin with, sounds, at different pitches and volumes, were sent through a speaker. The idea is that the audiologists watch for when your child reacts or turns towards the sound. There was a more advanced test which Oscar had never done before: every time they played a sound, Oscar had to put a man in a boat to show that he'd heard the noise. They'd asked me about doing this test before and every time I'd said that I didn't think he'd get the concept quickly enough and, if anything, he'd probably get too involved in wanting to put the men in the boat, so the test would be inconclusive. I said this again at the hearing test after his surgery. But the audiologist suggested we give it a go and just see. The long and the short of it was, as usual, when I underestimate him and tell myself something's too tricky, he goes right ahead and smashes it out of the park. There was absolutely no need for me to have underestimated him in this instance. The audiologist had started by helping Oscar, using her hand over his. When they heard the beep, together, they put the man in the boat. But then, just like that, having released her grip and left him to it, he did it all on his own. With varying pitches and frequencies being played, every time after that, he waited, paused for the sound and when he'd heard it, put the man in the boat. I was absolutely amazed by him. I talk about not wanting others to underestimate the capabilities of our kids a lot. How I want people to understand that although Oscar may be a man of few words at times, his understanding is all there. Because of this, I acknowledge it's easy to assume that he doesn't get stuff and to brush it off as too hard. But this was another reminder that Mummy sometimes gets it very wrong. The hearing test flagged up that he still had moderate hearing loss in one ear. It was the one the cholesteatoma had been in and the one they had inserted the titanium implant in, sadly. I say sadly because the operation and the implant obviously hadn't been that effective, which was deflating. He'd gone through so much to get to this point and still he had hearing loss. I wouldn't give up, though, believing there must be something else they could do.

Blog Comments – Thank You NHS

'We had gone in for our pre C-section chat and the midwife asked if I wanted anything specific on the notes. I said (holding back tears) I didn't want any negativity or anyone saying sorry when Max was born. That midwife started writing. However, another midwife who I hadn't even noticed was in the room, came over and looked me straight in the eye and said, "No one will say that he's your beautiful baby boy," then she just disappeared. I never saw her again. But her presence and words still provide me comfort today and I think of her often.'

Hayley Greenhill

'I was so distraught when the doctor confirmed Sienna's diagnosis and I'd felt like I was having an out-of-body experience. The doctor on HDU [High Dependency Unit] at the John Radcliffe in Oxford crouched beside me and took my hand. She then said to me, "I know that this feels like bad news right now, but I promise you your little girl will bring you more love than you ever thought possible." Her words are the only thing that sits strong in my memory of that day, it meant so much at a time when I was falling apart.'

Jacqui Hicklin

'I knew that there was a high chance that Rory would have Down syndrome, but I hadn't even heard of Hirschsprung's disease. At three days old, Rory developed sepsis and was given a stoma. He was in NICU for a very long time and was very poorly. One hard night one of the NICU nurses came over and held my hand and said, "I hope you realise that when you are here, he is your baby but when you can't be here, we care for him as if he is ours."'

Jayne Taylor

5

It Comes Down to Love

This particular day started at 4.25 a.m. for us. Oscar, having had another unsettled night, awoke and was apparently ready to start the day then. Thankfully, Chris got up with him and left me to have a lie-in, as I'd decided that it would be a good idea to go out for a few drinks and dinner with friends the night before, so was feeling really rather grateful that he'd stepped up so I could catch a few more zzzzs.

It was all going sooooooo well. A lazy breakfast together, the kids playing outside in the sunshine. It seemed a picture-perfect bank holiday weekend. That was, until Oz started throwing stones from our newly laid path, that we'd had put down the side of the house, all over our newly laid decking. Chris hadn't noticed this straight away, nor had he noticed Oscar finding an open drain (again, down the side of the house) and putting his hand and foot in it. But when he did, Chris, whom we'd all consider a cool, calm and collected type of guy, well, he just about lost his shit and there ended the morning calm. It was then that Chris decided that he needed to build a gate so that Oscar couldn't get access to the stone path, or the drain, and he decided that it absolutely needed to be done there and then or else (and I quote), 'We're going to spend the entire bank holiday weekend sweeping stones off the decking, Sarah.'

Anyone who knows us well will know that Chris has previous for 'doing jobs' at the most inopportune times. Whilst I'm scrambling around before a holiday – washing and packing clothes, tidying the house so it doesn't look like a bomb's gone off in it after we've left, all whilst entertaining and looking after three kids, invariably Chris is found outside washing the cars. If we're heading out for the day, depending on the season, he'll suddenly feel the need either to mow the lawn or to rake the leaves. Not to mention the time he used his paternity leave, just after I'd had Oscar and was in the depths of despair, to build borders in the garden. I appreciate I'm not painting him in the best of lights here, but at the risk of gender-stereotyping, having spoken to many, many friends about this, I'm sure I'm not alone.

Anyway, Chris then set off to buy the bits he needed from Wickes. While he was out, Alfie decided to stick a bead up his nose. Having never done this up till now, aged four (it's usually Oscar), Alfie went bat-shit crazy and the bead became lodged ever further up his nose. I tried in vain to recover the bead, now regretting the fact that I had gone out and drunk far too much Prosecco the previous night, as Alfie flailed around as if he'd been shot. Thankfully, Chris returned a few minutes later, managed to calm him down and get the bead out of his nose (see, he does have his uses sometimes). Although you might wonder what happened next. Well, Chris obviously set to, building his new gate. And me, Oscar, Alfie and Flo? Yeah, we drove thirty minutes up the road to a 'safe' park (and by safe, I mean gated, away from a main road and smallish in size so that I could keep a proper eye on all three kids) just to get out of the house and do something. I'd wondered if any of them might fall asleep on the way there and, luckily for me, they did. I obviously wouldn't be saying 'luckily' later when none of them would go to bed, but right then, sitting in that car park, in the middle of the Surrey Hills, listening to them snore their heads off, I was living the dream, guys.

* * * *

I'd found out that, just after I'd had Oscar, a family member was telling a 'friend' of theirs the news regarding his diagnosis. Their response went something along the lines of, 'Really? I'm so surprised Sarah's had a baby with Down syndrome. It's not as if she smoked during her pregnancy or that she's got a low IQ. She's a clever girl, isn't she?'

ACTUAL WORDS FROM SOMEONE'S MOUTH.

I'm hoping here that the large majority of people know that your level of intelligence has nothing to do with whether you have a baby with DS or not. (For the record, I have no idea what my IQ is. I got three A levels in Dance, Theatre Studies and Media Studies, didn't go to university and instead trained as a dancer. I think it's safe to say my IQ would be mediocre/distinctly average, but always good to hear someone thinks I might be clever.) As for smoking during pregnancy, they're right, I didn't, but even if I had done, there is no evidence to support the theory that if you smoke, you're more likely to have a baby with DS.

What I've learnt over the nine years of having Oscar, is that people say some ridiculous things. I've heard some corkers. A particular favourite of mine was when someone asked me, when Oscar was just a few days old, if I thought it was something I'd done late in my pregnancy that had caused this. I'm not sure what she was getting at exactly, but if eating too many Polos causes DS, watch out, my friends.

In October 2016, the actress Sally Phillips, who also happens to have a son, Oliver, who has DS, made a documentary, *A World without Down's Syndrome*, which challenged the misconceptions around the condition. On the back of that documentary, there was a lot written about whether it's fair to bring a disabled child into the world because what happens if you, as parents, die before your child and then it's left to their siblings to look after them. Chris and I have obviously thought about 'What happens if?' and, call me naive, but surely it's simple. Surely it comes down to LOVE?

And I'm not likening DS to an illness by any means (that would make me as bad as certain professionals in that documentary), but if ANY of my family members became poorly or needed me to care for them or look out for them, I would. Why? Because I love them. Simples. And I'm talking my mum, my dad, my sisters, nephews, nieces, whoever they were. You just would, surely? It's my hope that by the time I'm gone, Oscar will be living independently. Maybe that's optimistic? But even if he wasn't, and he needed extra care, we would put that care in place and would hope that his family would look out for him because that's what families do, isn't it? Not because they had to or felt obliged to. . . but because they love him and would WANT to look out for him.

We didn't have any decision to make about whether we brought a child with a disability into the world. We got what we were given. We did, however, make the very calculated and planned decision to bring Alfie and Flo into the world when we did. Not because we wanted them to 'care' for Oscar later in life, but because we knew that ultimately EVERYONE would benefit. Oscar for having them, but also them, for having him. When the debate becomes about, 'But what happens when the parents die?' although it's undeniably a factor to think about, I don't think it's a sufficiently valid reason not to bring a baby with DS into the world.

I judge nobody for their choices. We are all so very different after all. I understand women wanting to screen in their pregnancies and I understand those that don't. But after reading the message below, from a woman who'd just started following my social media page, it restored my faith that 'putting ourselves out there' and sharing our story (both the ups and the downs) had had a positive impact.

Dear Sarah

I found out a week ago I'm expecting my second child. I've spent each day sick to the stomach with worry, barely getting out of bed. I'm panicking, you see, as I turned forty last month. That's the danger age, isn't it? Where it all gets hard, and the babies are all poorly. I've called the hospital twice asking to make sure I get a scan in time to be screened. I've read the leaflet. Googled my options.

Then, just by chance, one of my friends liked something on your page and I read. I read and read and read some more. Dear God, what on earth have I been thinking? Why do I need screening? This baby is a miracle, even more so as I've spent twenty years desperately trying to conceive in the first place. I have jostled thoughts and ideas in my head and spent almost an hour trying to convince myself I was right and should push for my screening on time. Then I watched a video of Oscar. Thanks, Oscar, you've made up my mind for me. My little boy deserves to have the little brother or sister that we are being blessed with. I won't be screening anybody or anything. And I certainly won't be 'discussing my options'. This is our baby, and he/she is going to be loved.

I really love the boy's name Oscar so excuse me if I pinch it.

Much love to you and your wonderful and inspirational family

Anon

Through my page and in writing my blog, pretty much every week I am contacted by new mums and dads. I say 'new' because they've either just had a baby with Down syndrome or have been given a prenatal diagnosis that they're expecting one and the general feeling of the messages they send is of understandable fear of the unknown. When I receive such emails, I can only liken how they must be feeling to the way I felt back when I first had Oscar. I tell them it's okay to feel the things they do because every emotion we feel is real and that they mustn't feel bad for feeling that way. But then I received another message from a woman, who'd messaged me previously to tell me she's currently expecting a baby with DS, saying that she still hadn't come to terms with it and was really, really struggling. And it got me thinking about what's worse: knowing ahead of time or being like me. Perhaps if you know ahead of time you have an idea in your mind … and spend your pregnancy consumed with worry about how it's going to affect your family. Or, on the flip side, might it give you time to come to terms with everything and potentially start accepting the situation?

If, like me, you don't know ahead of time and had all these idealistic views about how life with a new baby would pan out and then DS was mentioned and all those hopes and dreams were quashed – or I THOUGHT they were – is that better? Although it was a shock and an adjustment, once I had Oscar with me, I couldn't not love him? I often wonder what the answer is. I often wonder, too, if I am the right person to 'talk' to these new mums and dads because everyone's experiences are so different, and acceptance can come for some people at very different stages. It's easy for me to sit here and say, 'Everything's going to be okay. You'll love this baby more than you ever imagined,' but sometimes I wonder if these new parents believe me.

Once, when Oscar and I were on our way in to London, waiting for the same train as us was a young man who I assumed was around twenty-five to thirty years old. He was with another man of roughly the same age. It was early on a Saturday evening and the pair were obviously heading in to London for a night out (I later spied some theatre tickets in one of the guy's hands). Nothing particularly different about two guys heading in to town together you might be thinking, except, on closer inspection, I realised that one of the men had Down syndrome. He looked cool. He was dressed much the same as the guy he was with. And I'm not sure if they were, but I got the impression they were brothers.

Oscar was happy watching the trains, so, trying my best not to act too much like a creepy stalker-type again, I spent the next few minutes watching the pair's interaction. The guy with Down syndrome (let's call him Sam) hadn't done his coat up all the way, so his brother (let's call him Matt) zipped it up for him. They then shared a long hug, when it looked as though neither of them wanted to let go. I felt a little emotional watching them, I guess because I automatically pictured Oscar and Alfie together like this later in life and hoped they'd share the same bond.

Next, Matt wandered away from Sam and then playfully hid from him behind a sign. Sam, clearly finding it amusing, followed him and quickly found him. They were playful. They were happy. But I couldn't help thinking that the interaction between them seemed almost childlike and, for some reason, I decided I didn't want to watch any more.

Shortly afterwards everyone boarded the train. Sam and Matt were sitting just a few seats in front of us. About ten minutes into the journey, I realised Sam had obviously got up to use the toilet. As soon as Matt heard the bathroom door open, he shot up out of his seat and shouted to Sam to come back, as he'd already started walking the opposite way to where his brother was sitting. Once we got to Waterloo, when Oz and I stood up to get off the train, I realised that Sam and Matt were behind us. The helping him with his coat, the hide-and-seek game at the station, the calling him back from the toilet because he hadn't remembered where his brother was – all of these showed me that Sam really needed his brother that day. Would Oscar always need us that way too? Did it matter if he did? But for some reason, it seemed to get to me that day. For the record, when I REALLY thought about it, Sam appeared to be having a great time. This was MY issue. Not at all Sam's, or even Matt's. I presume it's natural, though. To fear for our kid's future, I mean. I presume it's natural to look at people with DS just that bit further ahead in their lives and wonder what will become of our own child when they get to that age? What I do know is that when Oscar was a baby, imagining him at four-and-a-half would have been a scary prospect, but now we were here, four-and-a-half years on, it isn't in the least bit scary. Trying to predict how Oscar would be at twenty-five that day was too much for me. I didn't like looking TOO far ahead because somehow that felt more daunting.

Any time I've had a wobble in the past, and still to this day, Chris has always been the one to talk me down. He'll often remind me that, 'Fear and worry is just your mind, pre-empting something that hasn't happened yet and may never happen.' It's something he says that always helps me to rationalise my fears. For I know he's right. Why DO we spend time worrying about the future, when it's wasted time and energy? Living in the moment feels a lot less scary. Okay, so maybe that's two things he's good at. Calming me right down when I'm worrying about Oscar and what lies ahead AND getting beads out of our kids' noses. He might well be a keeper after all.

Blog Comments

'An NHS nurse turned to me in front of Sam and said, "What's wrong with him?" I feigned ignorance and said there's nothing wrong with my son. He may be non-verbal, but he can understand everything you say.'

@suzywriting

'I'd been on the phone with someone who worked in a special needs setting, and they'd said, "More often than not r*****ed children have slow parents".'

@321_mum

'A consultant told me I could move to Mongolia and then no one would notice the Down syndrome as, "Everyone looks like that there"!'

Angie David

'A churchgoing friend of mine blamed "The sins of the fathers" for my son having Down syndrome.'

Michele Coyle

6

Follow Your Heart

When Oscar was tiny, I remember watching the Christmas Marks & Spencer advert and there, amongst all the other gorgeous children modelling the clothes, was the most beautiful little boy who happened to have Down syndrome. He'd caught my eye as the camera panned to him, because his face had lit up and he'd looked like he was having the time of his life. I later found out his name was Seb, that he was five years old, and his mum Caroline ran a blog. From that day on, I was hooked (still am) and love reading about all of Seb's incredible achievements. At the time, watching him on that TV commercial, gave me, a first-time mum navigating her way through accepting her little boy's diagnosis, some hope. I looked at him that day and shared that television ad with all my family and friends to show them what was possible. (I realise now I spent a lot of time back then trying to prove to others all the things Oscar would be capable of. I felt like some sort of advocate for him, as if I had to prove his worth.)

Seb has always been my inspiration and I remember thinking that if Oscar was half as amazing as him, I'd be happy. Seb, along with a couple of other children who happen to have DS, were among some of the first who appeared in mainstream national media campaigns, and it was such a breakthrough for our community. So when, through my blog and social media page, Oscar was approached by a modelling agency, I was so chuffed. And then, shortly afterwards, when I found out that he'd been chosen to appear in an advertisement for Tesco's F&F Clothing range, I was thrilled.

Oscar had done a couple of modelling jobs previously. The first had been with Alfie and Flo for JoJo Maman Bébé. Oscar was about to turn four, Alfie was almost three and Flo was ten months old. It was boiling hot day, the shoot was in this gorgeous house in Kent and I'd enlisted the help of my best friend to come with me to help look after the kids, knowing that more than likely it would be carnage. The house was someone's actual home that the people making the ad had hired for the day. I was so conscious that the ornaments and low-level lamps were far too tempting for my kids not to touch that we watched them like hawks. Most of the shoot was done in the garden, much to the relief of both me and the JoJo Maman Bébé team, as I think we were all having heart attacks at the potential for accidents just waiting to happen. The kids did so well. Oscar and Flo seemed in their element. Alfie didn't love it as much but one of my favourite ever photos of him is of him sitting in a pair of PJs on the step of the little summer house, looking royally pissed off. It's a classic and one to bring out at his eighteenth. One of the biggest issues with kids modelling is that the brand is trying to capture them looking gorgeous, but also the clothing they're wearing in the best possible light. Whilst Oz was enjoying the camera, lots of the shots were of him sitting on a little bench. As he sat, he'd put his legs out in front and grab his top, looking all coy and cute, then they'd be continually having to straighten him out for the next shot. It was gorgeous and stressful in equal measure. But they got their shots in the end.

Oscar's second appearance in an ad was for Mac (as in Apple).

Oscar and I had travelled up to London the night before and the production company had put us up in a swanky hotel. When I'd said yes to Oscar doing the ad, I'm going to be honest with you, I was dubious as to whether he'd cope, as my main worry was that he wouldn't do as he was told. Also, as he'd got older, he was becoming more wary of new people and different surroundings. I can't tell you how nervous I was, wondering if I'd done the right thing. Staying in a hotel was a big change to his routine too. He'd been seen by wardrobe and make-up early on the morning of the shoot and we were driven to location with a handful of other children. The parents or chaperones were told to go into a different room, but they'd said that I could stay on set just in case Oscar got distressed (he was also the youngest by far), if I was out of sight.

Half-way through the shoot, one of the women from the production team came over and when I asked how he was getting on she said, 'He was being sooooooo good and so well-behaved.' I COULDN'T BELIEVE IT! Aside from the fact that I was just so happy that it had gone well, what I loved most about the day was that it seemed to me that Oscar was simply a part of a small group of kids and it wasn't at all about him being singled out as the token 'disabled' one. He was just one of a bunch of kids, having fun. There was nothing more to it than that. There have been days in the past, like when we've had to take him for an operation or got him fitted for his 'special' boots to help him walk or been swimming in the hydro pool with a bunch of other disabled kids, that I've felt sad for Oz. Sad that he's had to face different challenges to the next kid. I guess there've been times I've felt that life can kind of suck. But that day, I thought back to the first few weeks after he was born and the moments I've just described and felt so grateful for the opportunities Oscar has had, the life he's leading and how being a part of this little guy's life has made my life.

* * * *

As the day of the Tesco shoot approached, I'm not sure if I felt excited for Oscar and the opportunity or more anxious that he wouldn't do what he was told on the day. He was almost another year older now (nearly five years old) and I knew that he had developed much more of a bull-in-a-china-shop approach to everything. I'd been worried that Oz might be a bit too much.

I'd woken up in a right old mood that morning. The bad mood was mainly because I'd said yes to doing something that, in hindsight, I wished I hadn't. I do this all the time, you see, and it's one of the things that really annoys me about myself. However, the upside of this is that I sort of redeem myself in these situations, as I really don't like letting people down, so I end up doing whatever it is anyway (albeit in a huffy grump).

A few weeks prior to this, Oscar had been selected for a River Island casting. We'd driven all the way in to London on a Saturday afternoon, only for Oscar to flat out refuse to join in. I think I spent most of my time there trying to coax him off the floor, all the while assuring the photographer, his assistant AND the three ladies on the casting panel that this wasn't normal Oscar behaviour and that I really wasn't sure what had got into him today. Oscar, completely nonplussed, just sat there cross-legged, shaking his head in protest, refusing to budge. So, after the disaster of the casting, Chris and I had decided that perhaps modelling wasn't for Oz just now and we'd leave it for a bit. But then the modelling agency called and said that another client was looking for a child who happened to have Down syndrome, that they'd really liked the look of Oscar and if we didn't want to go to the casting, we didn't have to. After what had happened with River Island, I explained that Oscar always needs time to warm up to an idea and at a casting, where they whizz you in and out, it's never going to work for us. After they'd asked us to send a few more photos and a video clip of him instead, I honestly just assumed that, as they hadn't seen him in the flesh, we'd never hear from them again.

But Oscar got booked! So, when I woke up that morning, the day of the shoot, a feeling of dread came over me. WHY had I said yes? Would he even want to take part? Was he going to cause a scene? And would we be wasting everyone's time? Again.

We arrived and Oz was relaxed. When we got in to hair and make-up, however, he lost his s**t. I mean, he REALLY didn't want to do it. We thankfully got through that – with key bribery tool number one, the promise of watching the iPad – but when it came to his turn, he basically sat down and refused to budge. Deep down, I had a feeling that if he could watch one of the other children having a go, he would be more likely to try himself. I knew that giving Oz just that extra bit of time to get used to his surroundings – the lights, the sounds, the mass of people on set – that he could do it! So I asked them if they'd mind. They called another model onto the set and, gingerly, Oscar looked up, his curiosity having got the better of him. He watched with interest. And just like that, with a little help from an older boy who was also modelling, and beckoned him over, Oscar wandered up to his new friend, stood next to him and only went and pulled it out of the bag. I must say the team were all amazing. There was a guy working on set who caught Oscar's attention from the start. He was fab with him. He juggled oranges, got Oz to give him high fives, which he obviously found hysterical, and just generally made him laugh.

At the end of the shoot, the photographer turned to me and said that he'd done brilliantly and that they'd got some great images. I just loved that Oz was being photographed alongside his typically developing peers in a mainstream nationwide advertising campaign and that he'd held his own.

On day two, Oscar had been booked to wear one outfit, but after the success of the day before, they said they wanted him to stay on to model a second outfit. He went on for outfit number one with three other children and, again, did so well. At this point, standing to one side, I was thinking, 'Wow, buddy, you're really nailing this.' Juggling-oranges guy was there again (thank goodness!) and being just as great at his job as he had been the day before – he managed to get all four kids eating out of the palm of his hand (metaphorically, obvs). They were all absolutely loving him. So much so that having got them all hyped up into a frenzy for the 'We're all having so much fun together' group shot, when they then said they wanted some 'chilled' shots and asked the kids to stand still, the other three did, but Oz was having far too much fun to stay on one spot after all that excitement. After watching from behind my hands for a little while, my inner voice screaming something along the lines of, 'Oscar, seriously dude, you were doing so well, don't f**k it up now,' I suggested it might be a good idea if he had a few minutes of downtime. Obviously, being super-lovely, they agreed and, thankfully, after a few minutes on the iPad (key bribery tool number one used again) he did indeed calm right down.

But when they produced his second, and final, outfit of the day, and it was for a dress-up themed photo, Oz decided that enough was enough and was basically having none of it. Let's all remember here Oscar has never been the biggest fan of a costume and, at this stage of the game, they were reeeeeeally pushing their luck, so we decided collectively that we should quit while we were ahead and call it a day. Just before we left, one of the women who was running the day said they thought Oscar had done brilliantly and that they were all really pleased with him. And breathe.

I thought about Oscar's time on set afterwards, of how amazing it was that he had got the opportunity, and how great it was that a kid like him was being represented in mainstream media. But then I also thought that no matter how much we all try to convince ourselves the world has moved on and people like to see diversity, the truth is, when a child like Oscar's chosen, it's still a really frickin' big deal. I hope one day that it's not like that at all, that including a child like Oscar in an ad campaign is simply par for the course.

Around this time, although Oscar had had a great couple of terms at his school, Chris and I approached them about the possibility of his repeating reception the following year. It was something we'd been thinking about for several reasons. Since Oscar had started school in September, he had come on so much, both socially and developmentally.

When he'd first started at the school, getting him to sit down and focus on anything was a struggle. His communication book over recent months, however, had been full of how brilliantly he'd coped, working well alongside his peers and joining in with class activities.

There had never been any doubt in our minds that the school had been anything short of amazing with him, but there had always been that niggling feeling that repeating the year would be best for him to cement everything he'd learnt so far. We felt that if he was allowed to repeat the year, it would stand him in good stead to stay in a mainstream school for longer. Our first reason was that he'd been born in the summer (July), so was already young for his year group. His speech was obviously very delayed, although we were seeing developments all the time, and try as we might, toilet training just wasn't happening yet. All that, in addition to the fact that he had had a large chunk of time off in January and February to have his operation, recover and attend various follow-up appointments, made us feel that we should at least ask the question.

I was dubious about what the school would say, as I'd been told it's not usually the done thing for a child to repeat in this area (Surrey). They were concerned that he would be separated from his friends in his existing class, which we got, but we felt that although he might be sad initially, the reasons we had given would outweigh that concern. They said they'd be happy for him to move up to Year 1 because they would continue to put in place the support he needed, but once presented with the reasons we and Oscar's supporting professionals wanted to keep him back, they understood why we wanted to do this. Initially, I wasn't clear if it was the school or the local authority which would make the final decision, but it turned out that in our area and because the school was an academy the joint and final decision lay with the school governors and the headteacher.

We had to wait a few months for an answer, but, shortly before the end of the last term of Oscar's first year in reception, our request was approved. He could repeat the year.

I spent hours reading through the local authority's policy on this and found out that they could potentially ask Oscar to skip a year and catch up with his age-appropriate peers in the future if they wanted to. This was something that worried me slightly as the thought of him skipping a whole year of learning seemed ludicrous to me. Having done my research, however, I saw that the chances of this happening and of their having a viable reason for him to make that jump would be slim. I mean, seriously? Is there any child, regardless of having additional needs or not, who could make such a leap? So, I felt assured we were doing the right thing.

We had Oscar's annual review coming up and I asked if we could put in writing that Oscar would not at any point be asked to move up a year. We succeeded in having the point included in that year's review, but of course reviews are amended every year, so I wasn't at all sure that we'd succeed in future in keeping that point in. I knew there was a chance they could refuse and, later down the line, ask him to skip a whole year, but I kind of felt like that was a battle for another day or, as Chris would say, a battle that might not need to be fought. And by this point I'd learnt that, as a parent of a child with additional needs, I would just have to be ready for any battle that came along if it meant fighting for what my child needed and deserved.

I think some people thought we regretted sending Oscar to school when we had done. Other parents in a similar position defer their children starting school and give them another year in nursery or preschool, which we hadn't wanted to do. To make it clear, Chris and I didn't regret sending Oscar to school when we did. One thing I've realised in life, whether it's to do with our children or our own life choices, is that you've got to follow your heart, and ours was telling us, that for our Oscar, this was the right thing to do for him at this point.

It was July, the final month of Oscar's first year of reception and his first ever sports day. There was a crowd and I wasn't sure if he'd decide against being part of it all. But I'm not sure what I loved more about the morning in the end; it was either watching Oscar's teaching assistant's face, beaming with pride as she ran behind him, spurring him on as he crossed the finish line, or that I got to watch Oscar taking part, alongside his peers, in running races, throwing the javelin and discus, taking part in the high jump and hula-hooping, all with the biggest smile on his face. He absolutely loved it. I'd be lying if I said he got his form right in all the events, but that didn't matter to me. He did it, right? Another one of those moments that will stay with me for ever was him finishing the running race. He wasn't first, second or third; in fact, he came joint last with a little girl, who, to guess from her expression, felt the same way that I do about running. Painful, but what I won't forget was the support from his peers and their parents, all cheering him on from the sidelines, all right behind him. I like to think that, on that day, a few of the parents' preconceived ideas about what a child with DS looked like slipped away. I can't be sure, but I'm pretty sure they did.

Blog Comments – 'Looking back, what would you tell yourself and other parents in the same position. . .'

'. . . that every child with DS is an individual and will have their own strengths and weaknesses just like any child.'

Anon

'. . . not to cry, that it wasn't my fault and that once those first hard two weeks are over and your mind and life isn't in such chaos, that it will all settle down and you will get the chance to enjoy him.'

Nikki Jennifer

'. . . take one day at a time and not panic about the future. Our daughter Beth (twenty-two) has recently been signed by a modelling agency and we are having so much fun with it all. Beth has changed me so much for the better and we have met wonderful people that I never would have met in different circumstances.'

Fiona Matthews

'. . . to celebrate every step forward that their child takes. At times there may be tears and challenges, but their child will bring them more joy and love than they can possibly imagine. My child has done many things I wouldn't have the courage to do – horse-riding, canoeing, rock climbing, potholing, cycling from one side of England to the other and is a brilliant swimmer. Life didn't stop for us, it gave us the determination to push ourselves, to both study for degrees. Enjoy every precious minute. My son is now fifty-one.'"

Christine Holt

'. . . not why me but thank god me! Because I always believed he was given to me because I would always do the very best for him and I was grateful I was given the chance to be his mum. Those seven little words helped me in the beginning, but have helped every single day since, too.'

Anon

7

Play Date

It was the summer holidays and I found myself in France, sitting in a dark hotel room, waiting for Flo to drift off. Chris and the boys were up the hallway in another room (we couldn't get a family room) and I could hear the pandemonium unfolding as Chris tried to settle them and I sat, feeling grateful for my choices right then. We'd decided at the last minute that we would have a holiday after all. We were having an extension built on our house and, up until this point, we'd stayed in it, amongst the dust and rubble, with building going on all around us. But because they were screeding the floor, we had decided to escape to Chris's family's chalet in the Swiss Alps. We were on our way to Switzerland the following day.

Oscar had his first ever holiday to Switzerland when he was seven weeks old. Since then, because we are lucky enough to have family out there, we've holidayed at the chalet several times. And every time we do, Chris and I always comment on the way people react to Oscar. I'm not sure what or why it is, but we always notice an increased number of people staring at him.

We noticed it when we stopped in France, too, so it's not just Switzerland; and we're pretty sure it's not out of malice, rather that people are intrigued, though it can, at times, be very blatant.

Perhaps it's because at home we are more at ease with our surroundings. We know that in our village, nobody would really give him a second glance and, if they did, it would only be to say hi. Maybe it's because people with DS are more widely seen in and around London, where we live, than in the mountains of Switzerland. Who knows? But a few days in to our trip, when a woman was constantly staring at him, I made sure I distracted her by waving and shouting, 'Hiiiiiii,', so she knew I'd caught her. In hindsight, this was rather passive-aggressive of me, but she scurried off sharpish after that, so it did the trick. And, although nothing to do with DS, when we were at the lake, Oscar spotted a bucket he quite liked the look of that a little boy had been playing with in the water and went over and tried to pinch it. The little boy got cross with Oscar and started kicking the water up in his face. Not usually one to be backwards in coming forward, Oscar, as I watched this time, stood shocked, frozen on the spot. Just as I was about to step in and tell Oscar to move away from the little boy, who, rightly or wrongly, had only retaliated because Oscar had attempted to steal his bucket, I saw Alfie wade over, hands on his hips and start shouting at the boy: 'Stop splashing Oggar,' his name for Oscar, and then proceed to kick water in the little boy's face. I obviously stepped in at this point, but I couldn't help but smile. We've never once told Alfie that he needs to look out for his brother, even though it's something that Chris and hoped would evolve over time, but Alfie stepped in completely of his own accord because he wanted to protect his brother. And even though in this instance it wasn't about Oscar having Down syndrome, I figured Alfie felt the same in-built desire to protect his brother that Chris and I feel towards Oscar, when someone stares so obviously at him.

After this, both Oscar and Alfie continued playing in the water. I probably should have explained to Alfie that just because someone lashes out at Oscar or him, it doesn't mean that he has to retaliate. But I didn't. I asked Chris if he'd seen and when he said yes, we just smiled a knowing smile. Sometimes things are better left unsaid.

On the final day of the holiday, the one and only day it poured with rain, and I mean *torrential* rain, we'd decided to take the kids on a ride up the mountain in a cable car. We'd been expecting idyllic views, but instead we got wind, rain and ratty kids. The cable car cost us 90 Swiss francs (£70!!!!) and because of the rain and low cloud, we literally couldn't see a thing. Oz sat on the floor of the cable car pretty much the entire time because he was scared and Flo had done a poop in her nappy, so, as you can imagine, we were all massively regretting our choice of a confined space. Our friends who'd come out to Switzerland to stay with us had a little boy, who decided, at the exact moment the cable car set off, that he needed a pee. Despite our attempts to persuade him to do so into a nappy/disposable nappy bag/empty water bottle, he was having none of it and, moments later, his dad was seen holding him up by the window, willy out, hoping he'd pee into the wind (he got stage fright so couldn't do it in the end). When we got to the top of the mountain, the only place to grab a coffee and escape the weather was a brand-spanking-new restaurant with Dom Perignon umbrellas outside it. I'm not sure they appreciated five kids climbing on and off their bar stools and moving tables around for them, but that's holidays with kids, right?

When I had Oscar, one of the things I was worried about was, would we still be able to go on holiday like everyone else. Whilst there's the issue of insurance potentially costing more than a typical child – particularly if your child has health complications – like so many of my worries it has proved largely unfounded. Although going on holiday with Oscar has meant we haven't been able to relax as much as we might have done without him – because with a child like Oz we're always on high alert, wondering what he's going to get up to next – over the years things have got easier. We're still not quite at the stage where we could let him wander off alone at the swimming pool and we're still, nine years on, chasing him up and down the water slide, but he doesn't charge about half as much as he did when he was younger, and there are moments of calm. I'm often contacted by parents of little ones with DS who are around four or five years old, who feel exasperated, frazzled and just generally worn out. Their kids are a handful and it's exhausting. They ask me when it stops. I always say that we found Oscar the trickiest when he was four or five years old. He was no longer a toddler who we could scoop up and pop in the buggy if need be. At that age, he was fast, but with no sense of danger; that was tough for a while. I'm not sure I can pinpoint the exact moment it got easier, and, believe me, even now, I would say I'm always on my guard, pre-empting what Oscar's next move might be. But as Oscar has grown older, he has developed a better awareness of danger, also a desire to be like his brother and sister and to get things right. I'm not saying that when I give him an inch, he doesn't try to take a mile, but, over the years, although we might not yet be at the 'peruse the rails of Zara together, pick out outfits and have a chat' stage (the way the mother with a ten-year-old son with

DS was when I saw them all those years ago) I think we're getting there. Slowly.

Something that didn't even occur to me when I had Oscar was 'toileting issues'. And here we are nine years on, with the benefit of what I know now, and I can honestly say, 'It's been a journey.' With the benefit of hindsight, I wish I'd given him more credit. The advice, which I'm ashamed to say I dismissed, feeling that Oscar would have no concept or understanding of what was entailed, was to start kids with DS on the potty/toilet as soon as they can first sit up. I disregarded this advice because, to my mind, Oscar simply wasn't ready. But the general feeling now is that the sooner you can encourage them to sit on the loo, the better the chances of them being successful.

Towards the end of those summer holidays and with Oscar now five, I thought it was about time to give toileting a good go. We'd been putting Oz on the toilet before his bath to get him used to it, but, as yet, he hadn't 'performed'. I had been so hopeful that he'd go back to school dry and held onto the hope that, if we persevered, we'd get there.

It wasn't even 8 a.m. the morning after I'd made the decision and toilet training had commenced. I had the toilet door wide open, ready to whizz him in there. There was a toilet seat with handles and a step for him to step up onto the loo so that he'd feel safe and secure, allowing his feet to be flat on the floor with his knees in line. I'd read that going straight to the loo, instead of using a potty, would be ideal, as then you wouldn't have to transition from potty to loo – yet another hurdle. At this stage I had read much on the topic and also garnered a lot of advice from those who had walked this path previously. On the advice of my friend Karen, whose little boy, Lance, who also has DS, was just a few months older than Oz and who'd nailed it by now, I'd got myself an egg-timer, and kept setting it every twenty minutes so that I'd remember to take him.

So there we were, me with my egg-timer, Oz walking around pantless and so far he'd already peed on the floor twice, much to Alfie and Flo's disgust. We'd had a minor breakthrough in that before this time he wouldn't even have entertained sitting on the loo, but now it seemed he would. But there had still been no pees or poops in there. Now, I'm no quitter – except maybe around 3.30 p.m. on a Monday afternoon when I reach for the chocolate Hobnobs, having declared when I woke up that, 'This is it. I'm only going to eat healthy food for the rest of my life.' However, having started toilet training at 7.45 a.m. that morning, an hour and a half into it, it dawned on me that I'd already cleaned up seven wees on the floor and one, rather large, poop off the sofa.

Chris, who was on holiday that week and who is quite possibly one of the most anal people you could ever meet, had a fit over the possibility that Oscar might pee on our new extension floor. So one argument later, with me doing that whisper-shouty-type thing so the kids couldn't hear, along the lines of, 'Do you want to be wiping his arse when he's forty-three?', we decided it might be best if we confined Oscar, and his brother and sister, to the front room and downstairs loo, where the flooring was, at that stage, rubbish.

Although we were being kept entertained by the delights of *Paw Patrol*, *Fireman Sam* and *Andy's Dinosaur Adventures*, by lunchtime and copious amounts of wee later, I was losing the will to carry on, so we changed tack. I knew when to admit defeat. We tried the potty instead. We tried putting him in pants so that he'd feel that he was wet, rather than leaving him to go commando. And aside from cocking his leg in the air when he felt the wee trickle down his leg, he couldn't have cared less that he was now wandering around in wet pants. By this point, we tried lots of praise when he sat down because for the most part, he flat out refused to sit down on either the loo or the pott. And even though I had a whole packet of chocolate buttons in my pocket, ready to reward Oscar, he didn't hit the jackpot even once!

So, I gave up. Which I know sounds defeatist. I know that some would say, 'But you need to keep on trying. You need a run of at least three or four days when you can stay home and just go for it; Rome wasn't built in a day. . . blah blah blah,' but in all honesty, he was now getting very cross and causing a pretty big stink in the process. Quitting, and simply leaving it for a while, felt like the right thing to do.

And while I know we can't compare Oscar's development to that of Alfie and Flo, except as a mother of a child with DS and two kids who don't have additional needs, back then, I would compare them, to a much greater extent. Alfie took to toilet training so fast. I think maybe he had three accidents and then he was dry, day and night. Flo took a bit longer, but when we trained her, we felt she understood what was expected of her. Oz, at this point, appeared as if he couldn't have given less of a f**k!

The general feeling was that we'd failed – more me than Oscar, of course – but we did, on the plus side, come away from the experience having learnt some valuable life lessons:

1. Chris and I, much like when he's driving on the motorway and I'm navigating, do not do well as this

kind of team. . . Things go much more smoothly when he's at work.

2. Oscar may not have had success with his peeing and pooping, but he was on it with the Domestos spray and kitchen roll and became a dab hand at cleaning.

3. The brown sofa in our living room, which I had been hoping to replace because it was dated and old, was a godsend when it came to disguising stains.

Every cloud, right?

The toilet training journey didn't end there. It got better. Just consider this a brief pause in proceedings as we did get there in the end. I'll come back to this shortly.

Just after Oscar went back to school and into his second year in reception, he was invited on his very first after-school play date. It may sound a little silly to some of you, but an actual play date after school in our little world then was kind of a big deal. Oz was usually exhausted by the end of a school day and understandably not always at his best so, to be honest with you, it wasn't ever something I'd encouraged.

The previous year, he'd been invited on a play date which I'd ended up politely declining. Looking back now, I think this was because, although I knew he was liked, I worried a lot about his behaviour in someone else's house. He had this habit back then of continually wanting to go upstairs in someone else's home, get into their bed and would invariably end up throwing the duvet down the stairs. At school I knew he was being watched. I knew there'd be limited trouble he could get up to, being in a controlled environment. But his having free rein in someone else's home filled me with dread, so I did everything I could to avoid these social situations. The other reason that I never encouraged a play date was that he would need me there with him. And, with me, came two other little people – Alfie and Flo!

However, this particular time, the mother of a little girl in Oscar's class offered to have us round for a play date and dinner. My first instinct was to decline, telling her that it would be too much and that she didn't need all of us descending on her, but she was insistent and, in a moment of weakness, I accepted her invitation.

You've probably worked out by now that I have a habit of fearing the worst, catastrophising everything, so that if things *do* go well, it's always a lovely surprise. If they *don't*, then I feel like my expectations have been managed and there's no need for me to feel any kind of disappointment. It's a self-preservation thing, I think. It works for me, but is probably annoying for anyone around me listening to my wobbles. So you can imagine my delight in this instance when, having accepted the invitation, it turned out to be the best thing I could have done.

Oscar, Alfie and Flo all played beautifully and had a lovely time. They sat and ate their dinner, probably better than they would have done at home and when the little girl and Oscar went upstairs to play together, even though I felt a twang of panic – 'What if he starts throwing her toys around, breaks something, pulls off the duvets or plays too roughly with her' – I let him go.

It took everything in my power not to stop them and tell them to play downstairs where I could keep an eye on them. But I didn't. And the reason? Because there was a part of me that knew that sometimes you've got to give your children the benefit of the doubt. But it was also because the little girl's mother had given me a look that said it really was okay. I could see that she got it, that she understood, and she put me completely at ease.

So, we left them to it. At various intervals, they came downstairs as apparently they were 'moving house' and Oscar was 'off to work'.

After a little while, it had all gone a bit quiet, so I went up to check on them. As I approached the bedroom, I could hear the little girl talking to Oscar, giving him a running commentary of what they were doing and asking him the odd question here and there. And when I paused at the doorway, I saw them sat on the floor together, both dressed in hats and various other additional items of clothing, bags packed, with Oscar in charge of what looked like a toy pet carrier. They'd obviously just arrived at their new home. It probably doesn't sound like a big deal to most, but I could see how much Oz was enjoying it. I have spent so much time watching him over the years, always making sure that he wasn't up to something because I'd never wanted to come across as that parent who isn't on it, then it all goes to pot. But seeing them like that really made me smile. It taught me that, despite my reservations, sometimes, the things that seem like a bad idea at the time turn out to be really frickin' wonderful.

Being grateful to the little girl's mother reminded me of other people I was grateful to. Having walked out of the hospital with Oscar, still feeling a bit shell shocked about his diagnosis and his traumatic entrance into the world, I didn't really have the energy or foresight to say a proper thank you. I wasn't really thinking straight, but one of the people I would have loved to have said a huge thank you to was Jessica, the midwife who was looking after me the night Oscar was born. She was monitoring both Oscar and me as, at my routine forty-week check-up earlier that day, I had been sent to my local hospital because they'd found Oscar's heart rate was a bit slow and wanted to keep an eye on him. Fast forward to a few hours later and Oscar's heart rate had dropped dangerously low. It was so low that Jessica had pressed the alarm, and I'd been rushed off to have an emergency C-section under general anaesthetic.

It was the birth of my first son, sadly also the most traumatic experience of my life to date. I was scared. Chris wasn't allowed to stay with me in surgery and I will never forget the number of medics, working at such speed, to get me into theatre. I went into shock and couldn't stop shaking, but, in the moments leading up to me going under, I remember Jessica vividly – how calm she was, how professional and how very caring.

A year after Oscar had started school and four years after I'd started writing my blog, my in-box pinged.

I've literally just come across your blog and have spent a long time browsing your posts. I was the midwife who called the emergency bell the night Oscar was born. I remember the whole evening clearly as I had only just qualified as a midwife. His heart rate dropped for a few minutes, and I called the emergency bell and then he improved for a short while before dropping his heart rate again. The paediatric doctors were there for delivery, and I remember taking Oscar from the surgeon to the resuscitaire and feeling so relieved that he was crying and well. I have loved being able to see pictures of him doing so well all these years on and it's lovely to see what a gorgeous boy Oscar has grown to be. He was just the sweetest little baby boy.

As a midwife there are so many things that I will take
and learn from your blogs.

Wishing you and your family lots of health and
happiness, Jessica (Oscar's midwife)

I had never had the chance to say a proper thank you
to Jessica, but now I did. Reading her message, I could
feel my eyes stinging with tears. All these years later and
we were back in touch. I had my memories of what had
happened that night, but to hear her take on it gave me
huge comfort. Over the years, for many different reasons,
Oscar and I have met the most incredible team of NHS
doctors and nurses. Their kindness has never gone
unnoticed and when I think back to Oscar's birth and
the days that followed, those people who looked after us
will always have a very special place in my heart. Even
the paediatrician who apologised for Oscar's diagnosis;
I must thank her, too. The safe delivery of Oscar for a
start, his care afterwards. But the impact of her words that
night, her attitude and demeanour, have changed my path
for ever. Along with Oscar, she was the one who ignited
the fire in my belly to start writing. To share our lives and
gently educate. She has taught me so much about how
powerful our words can be and how treating others with
empathy and kindness should be our number one priority.
Had it not been for her, I wouldn't have started the blog,
my writing, had my books published or started training to
be a counsellor. I actually have so much to be grateful to
her for.

When Chris, Oscar and I walked out of the hospital ten
days after Oscar had been born, Chris asked my mum to
take a photo of us walking out of the exit. For the past
ten days, I had spoken about how I just wanted us to be

like everyone else, walking out of the hospital with my baby in a car seat. For it seemed to me at the time that, for everyone else, walking out of the hospital with their newborn baby had been no big deal at all. They seemed so nonchalant. So unfazed. But to me, right then, it meant everything. I still have that photo in a frame and from time to time I look at it. It will always be a reminder of such mixed emotions and of the incredible care we received back then.

Blog Comments

'My almost six-year-old has spent the better part of this past year conquering toileting. We've tried many times over the last 3–4 years, but it only clicked for her when SHE was ready. When she could feel and control what was going on. Up until then I really was just banging my head against a brick wall because NOTHING WORKED.'

Kelly Parry

'It was a long process for us. We started training Lana the summer before she started school. It took a week to make any progress at all. For a long time, it consisted of just adding it to Lana's routine and taking her at certain times throughout the day as she would rarely ask to go. School did the same. I still must remind her to go now at times and she's nearly eight. I do think she only gets the feeling when her bladder is full. Although she will take herself now. We are still to crack night times.'

Emma Kirk

'Robert is ten and we are still struggling with toilet. We do timed toilet. Trying to make it more of a routine. He is very good at pooing down toilet. He will pee but he still pees his nappy.'

Nelson Jacks

8

We Are All Different

*'Not being able to speak is not the same as not having
anything to say. It means you will need to listen to me
with more than just your ears'*

Unknown

With Oscar at school and Alfie at preschool, I had an
appointment with the nurse at my local community
hospital. Flo had come with me and the nurse that morning
was being particularly chatty. As the appointment went
on, we covered a few topics, but somehow, and I can never
really remember how these things pan out, we had got
onto the subject of Oscar. In the beginning, I'd often drop
the fact that Oscar had DS into conversations, but did
so less often as time went on. But we were talking about
toilet training and Oscar and his DS came up. At the time
it was mentioned, nothing more was said, but some time
later the nurse very gingerly asked, 'So your little boy with
Down's?. . . Is he?. . . You know. . . Is he bad?'

This sort of question often baffles me. When he was
super tiny, a friend of a friend asked me if there were any
early indications of how, and I quote, 'mentally retarded

he was going to be'. That had come as a shock. I couldn't believe people were still using 'mentally retarded' as an expression, and hoped it was down to her lack of education on people with learning difficulties, rather than complete and utter ignorance in general.

But this time, this person's words got to me. Mainly because she was a nurse, a medical professional, who, I assumed, given her age, would have had a wealth of experience, and here she was, standing in front of me, a mother, asking me how 'bad' my child's disability was. So, here's the thing, just something I should clear up: I find it insulting if people ask if a child who happens to have DS is 'bad'. I get why people ask: because they want to label him as mild, moderate or severe. They want to know where he is on the spectrum, because perhaps it makes them feel better to know. But it's a bit like me asking someone if their child needs extra support in an area at school or if they're clever. You just don't ask that sort of thing. Or that's how it feels to me at any rate.

And while I appreciate that, sure, there are some children with DS who are probably more high-functioning than others: that some children can talk, others not; some children are toilet trained early, for some it takes a bit longer; some are brilliant football players, and some are unlikely to play. In much the same way, some adults who happen to have DS work and others aren't able to; they are all very different. Much like you and me, I don't doubt.

The whole, 'Well Oscar doesn't look like he's got it bad,' which we've had on a few other occasions, is just so irrelevant. He has Down syndrome. You can't just have a 'little bit of Down's'. You either have DS, or you don't.

I thought this was worth mentioning because this nurse was lovely, and I didn't want to put her on the spot and embarrass her. Instead, I changed the narrative. I asked if she meant how was he getting on and, in the same breath, I told her that he was doing well, thank you.

A few short weeks later, Oscar had an appointment with his community paediatrician and, in the interests of keeping it factual, though I'm not sure if this has any relevance, I should point out that he was a locum, someone we'd never met before. We covered the various health-related stuff, but when we discussed Oscar's ongoing disrupted sleep, before I'd had a chance to finish, he said, 'Well, of course, "normal" children can have sleep issues too.'

Another example of a highly trained medical professional leaving me with very little doubt that, however clever they may appear in the eyes of society, some have ZERO emotional intelligence. For this doctor was essentially referring to my little boy as 'abnormal' or not a normal child. And I mean, REALLY?

When I was at school, there was nobody with additional needs in our class. In fact, there was nobody really any different to the whole heap of other Caucasian five- to eight-year-olds in our small village primary school. Oh, I tell a lie, there was one little boy who'd 'come over in a boat', as he was a refugee from Vietnam (showing my age there) but that was a big old deal at the time.

And although Oscar may have been the only one in his class and, in fact, his school, with Down syndrome I loved that when you looked around, although he was in a very similar local village primary school to the one I'd been in, there was 'difference' everywhere within our community. There were several other children with varying additional needs, different ethnic origins, different religions and children for whom English was a second language.

When Oscar started at school, I remember that one of my biggest worries was that the other children in his class would wonder why Oscar didn't say too much. But I was told that there were some children who were quieter than others, some who were louder, some who were gregarious and some who were very introverted. I was assured that Oscar's speech being limited probably wouldn't even occur to them, for all of them were different.

And then I received a message from a reader of my blog. It reminded me again just how lucky our kids are to be surrounded by 'different' every day. And how it seems that Oscar (and others like him) are silently influencing as they go. . .

I have met a number of moms lately who have children with DS, and I always ask them questions – I am amazed how they are changing the face of DS by sending their kids to mainstream schools etc., and hopefully thus the world will be educated to the possibilities and endearing qualities that these children have. Ignorance leads to stupid comments. Hurtful comments. But continue to educate all who cross your path. See negative comments as an opener to such conversations. I wish I knew more, and I hope my boys will come to know children with DS so that they can be better people themselves. I always say that the world would be an awful place if we were all the same. Difference (in all forms) is wonderful. It is not something to fear. Xxx

Walking home from school when Oscar was in his second year of reception, I'd always ask if he'd had a good day. And without fail, he'd always say, 'Yes.' I'd then say something along the lines of, 'Did you play with your friends?' And again, he'd always say, 'Yes.' I might walk a little further down the road and ask if he'd seen Mrs * (one of his TAs) and he'd always say, 'Yes,' usually with a big smile on his face because he loved her.

I'm not going to lie, the conversations were always a little one-sided. Aside from the odd 'banana' or 'park', because he was hoping I'd have a banana in my pocket or because he wanted to stop at the park on the way home, 'Yes' was probably his standard response to most questions. Oscar could understand a lot of what we were saying and could say a number of single words by now, but it seemed we were still quite far off having an actual conversation.

I'd often watch some of the other parents chatting freely with their kids – and don't get me wrong, I know most of them don't get that much out of their children after a day at school – but it was at times like these that I might occasionally feel a little sad that Oz and I couldn't converse in the way everyone else appeared to be doing. I so wished he could have told me what he'd been up to or who he'd played with, but, back then, it was just that bit too much for him.

But one day as we both got in the car (we were on our way to preschool to collect Alfie and Flo, who had a slightly later pick-up time than Oz) to make conversation, I asked him who he had seen that day. And when I listed all his teachers and TA's names, to my surprise, he attempted to say them all. And then when I said, 'Oscar, what did you play at school today?' – just to mix it up a little, you know, the whole 'Yes/No' thing can get a little tedious for everyone involved – he said and signed, 'Ball.'

I looked at him for a second, wondering if he had actually played with a ball or if he was making it up. He may even have been trying to appease me, to make me shut up, which, let's face it, would have been fair enough.

'You played ball, Oscar?' I asked.

And he said, 'Yes,' and then the name of the TA he had played ball with.

Proud enough that he'd been able to have a mini-conversation with me, I didn't really think much of it. Until a bit later, when I was reading through the entry in his communication book that day. His private speech therapist had written how his session had gone that morning. The TA he had in the mornings had written what he'd been up to earlier in class and then the final entry, that had been written by the TA that he'd mentioned by name earlier, went like this:

'This afternoon we shared a book together as well as matching some objects to the letter and sound 'a'. We also went outside, where we played ball, throwing and catching to each other and hitting it along the floor with a tennis racket.'

It may not sound much and, to be honest, it wasn't even the words that were that impressive, but I just loved that he'd remembered what he'd done AND was able to tell me who he'd done it with. It might be a long time before we can talk freely about the state of the FTSE 100, but it's a start, right? (Even if Oscar *could* talk, *I* wouldn't have a clue what he was going on about anyway.)

* * * *

One morning, in a very busy Sainsbury's, we managed to upset two people. I say busy, as apparently the whole world happened to be in our local supermarket, just as I whizzed in with three children in tow. We'd managed to park in a disabled bay and as we came out, as I had both Alfie and Flo in the trolley and Oscar was walking beside me, I decided to put Oscar in the car first in the interests of his safety. I then started to put the other two in, one at a time, when a woman in a car, whom I'd noticed had pulled up next to us, wound down her window and proceeded to shout, 'Excuse me, this space is for disabled people, you know!'

Taken off guard, I told her that my son, whom I'd already put in the car, was disabled, so we were allowed to park there.

Rolling her eyes at me, which I took as her not believing a word I'd said, she continued looking cross as she drove off.

I'm imagining she either hadn't seen Oscar – and looking at me, Alfie and Flo, assumed that none of us looked 'disabled', whatever that may look like – or she *had* seen Oscar walking to the car with us, but perhaps hadn't noticed that he had Down syndrome and so decided that none of us looked like we were eligible for a disabled badge? To make it clear, although Oscar could walk competently, he had, and still has, a disabled badge for a couple of reasons – he had no sense of danger and would often dart off at speed without thinking about the consequences. Being as close as we could be to the shops or the school helped me immeasurably. Sometimes he would tire easily so, again, being close to where we needed to get to made a big difference. Especially if he'd decided to sit and not budge, as we'd then have to carry him. Basically, he had a badge because he *is* disabled, and having a designated space for people like him helped us out massively. Also, aside from not needing to justify ourselves, I'm not sure who she thought she was to assume that none of us was disabled? What does someone with a disability even look like, remembering that not all disabilities are visible.

The other person we'd managed to royally pee off was an elderly gentleman in the shop itself, whom Oscar had whacked full pelt on the bottom. I'm not even going to try to sugar-coat this because it was a phase Oscar went through for a while when he was around three years old and was very intentional; he knew a whack on the arse would get a reaction. He would be trying to get your attention, you see. And in the main, when this happened, most people looked a little shocked initially and then they looked down at him and either smiled or said, 'Hi.' But this gentleman was visibly annoyed. And before I'd even had a chance to apologise, he turned round to Oscar, looked him square in the eyes and called him 'a very naughty boy'. And whilst to some, he may have been, a little bit of understanding on the gentleman's part wouldn't have gone amiss.

After I had Oscar, I'd always hoped I'd be lucky enough to have at least one, maybe two, more babies. Not just because I'd always imagined and hoped we'd be a big family, but also because it really felt important to me that Oscar should have a brother and/or sister in his life who could look out for him if ever he needed it – in much the same way, I figured, that they would all look out for one another. Now I'm not saying that they didn't all fight like cats and dogs sometimes. They'd get cross and I'm not going to deny the frequent slam-dunking of one another from time to time; yes, even demure, petite Flo would give as good as she got, I promise you. But seeing them together and the kindness they often showed to one another, and still do, well, it makes me beam.

One afternoon, after school, when Oscar was five and Alfie was four, they were all playing in the garden. Oscar was being quite vocal and I could see him and Alfie talking to one another out there. After a while, Alfie, who'd begun to look quite confused at his brother's ramblings, came running inside and said, 'Mummy, what did Ogger say? I don't understand him.'

Trying desperately hard not to say, 'Join the club, mate, I seriously have no clue half the time either,' I said something along the lines of, 'Don't worry, he's probably just trying to tell you about his day.'

Alfie looked at me, smiled, and ran back into the garden, and I heard a little voice say, 'Don't wowwy, Oggar, shall we go on the trampoline?'

'Oggar' smiled, and off they went.

What I loved is that Alfie didn't make fun of Oscar, he didn't call him out on it, he simply accepted him for who he was. Kids really don't see difference and, if they do, they just smile and get on with it. Exchanges like this one, whether it be between Oscar and Alfie, Oscar and Flo and even Alfie and Flo, remind me that kindness can go a long way. The elderly guy in the shop might have been having a bad day, he might have missed that Oscar had DS and should therefore, in my opinion, be given a little extra time to figure things out, e.g. that whacking people on the arse is definitely not cool. But that man didn't show him any kindness in any form that day, and I wonder if perhaps the younger generation have a thing or two to teach the older?

A few weeks earlier, when I wasn't looking, Oscar found the tic tacs in my car and proceeded to stick one up his nose. I only knew this because he was pointing to his left nostril and making weird dog-like sniffs. Thankfully, it came out after one big exhale through the nose – I obviously had to demonstrate – but, after the initial panic, it got me thinking about how I'd wanted so badly for him to be a typical baby when I'd first had him. How I'd willed and wished him to be 'normal' for quite some time afterwards. And it got me thinking, there'll never be a dull moment with 'different', will there?

Blog Comments

'A woman I didn't know chatted to me asking questions about my baby. When I mentioned he had DS she started calling him an "it". That was my cue to end the conversation!'

Lisa Briggs

'When speaking to a SENDCO [special educational needs and/or disabilities coordinator] at a prospective secondary school, he asked what my daughter's disability was. I told him it was Down syndrome, to which he replied, "Oh, we haven't had one of *them* before!." The conversation went downhill from there and we didn't apply for a place.'

Tara Gool

'The very worst thing ever said to me was, "So will he die before you?" I mean there's healthy interest in learning more about DS and then there are deeply hurtful questions!'

@tattyloulou

9

'He's Not a Poster Boy For Down Syndrome'

'Sometimes we are tested. Not to show our weaknesses, but to discover our strengths'
Unknown

Back in January, Oscar had an operation to remove a cholesteatoma, a growth in his ear, and just before Christmas, he had another operation to check if it had grown back. His consultant had said in his pre-op assessment that if it hadn't grown back, it'd be a forty-minute procedure, but if it had, it'd take about two hours.

Just over four hours later, he came out of surgery. . .

The good news was that the cholesteatoma hadn't grown back in the left ear; in fact, it had all healed so well that they'd had to drill through the mastoid bone again, which they hadn't expected as they thought it'd still be healing. This was one of the reasons the operation had taken so long and why Oscar looked like Mr Bump post-surgery, with a massive bandage around his head, but, all looked clear and cholesteatoma-free. However, while Oscar was under, out of curiosity, I'd asked the doctors to check that the grommet in his right ear was still in place. It wasn't, and whilst they'd been fitting another grommet, they'd found cholesteatoma had started spreading in *that* ear instead. We were told to come back to the clinic in two weeks' time so that they could attempt to take the sponge packing out, without a general anaesthetic this time. They said that they would carry out surgery to remove the new cholesteatoma early in the new year.

It wasn't the news we'd been hoping for. It was going to mean more check-ups and more procedures, which were likely to be ongoing now for years, but one thing that had always stood out for us in times like these was how strong Oz really was. He literally never let anything like this faze him, and we couldn't have been prouder of him that day.

I will say, though, that he has always hated having any observations done – blood pressure, temperature, SATS etc. He still refuses to wear a gown or to be taken down to theatre on a bed. Instead, he likes to walk down to surgery – the bed, the nurse, the hospital porter and me all in hot pursuit because he knows exactly where he's going. He walks through the entire hospital completely unfazed, struts into the holding area where a whole team of nurses, theatre staff, anaesthetists and others are stood around and, in true Oz style, he totally works the room, shouting, 'Hiya,' to them all. I mean, could he have been less fussed? It was one of those moments that made me smile and blub in equal measure. It was so lovely to watch, but I don't think there is anything worse than watching your baby, however old they are, go under for surgery.

Shortly after the bombshell of more cholesteatoma, Oscar and I travelled to the Royal Brompton Hospital in London for his annual heart check-up. When he was ten months old, he had open-heart surgery to repair a VSD [ventricular septal defect] in his heart. On this day, in true Oscar style once again he wasn't the most co-operative of patients as, although he's fairly laid-back most of the time, as I've said above, he hates any kind of observation and the sight of doctors and nurses can send him into a fit of rage. And in true Sarah style, on this day I let my guard down again – I really should learn never to do that – because they found that Oscar has raised pulmonary artery pressure and although he is showing no symptoms – he's not out of breath, doesn't tire easily – this could be caused by either the heart or the lungs. The VSD closure, thankfully, looked good, but he has a leaky valve, so this could be why his pressure was raised *or* it could be that his lungs are under strain, either because of sleep apnoea or aspiration.

They said they'd get him back to the Brompton for an overnight sleep study at some point the following year and book him in the next day to have an ECHO/ECG under sedation so they could have a proper look at what's happening. It felt like a bit of a punch when you're already down after the previous week and his ear, to be honest. I mean, seriously, could this kid get a break any time soon? But hey, they were monitoring him and he was in the safest of hands, so we just tried to stay positive.

It could have been the tingly arrival of my friend the cold sore, the little friend that rears its ugly head about every six months, usually around the same time that my lovely dad exclaims, 'You must be suffering with exhaustion, Sar.' It could be the cold and cough that I was slowly getting over or the long list of things I was yet to do before Christmas was upon us. But I felt so flippin' frazzled.

Obviously, the news about Oscar's cholesteatoma returning and the pulmonary hypertension kind of knocked us sideways, but it was all the other things that were supposed to happen at this time of year that added to the frying of my already fried brain.

Red tops and Santa hats I was supposed to have sourced for Alfie and Flo's Christmas performance, the Christmas shopping I was only about a quarter of the way through and the pile of wrapping I was yet to tackle. A mental note to remember sausage rolls and a change of outfit on Monday for Oscar's reception Christmas party, not to mention presents for his TAs, which I hadn't even thought about yet. Food and drink shopping for various guests we had coming over between Christmas and New Year; emails that had been hanging around in my in-box for weeks that I had yet to reply to; deadlines I was trying desperately hard to meet, but failing to; girls' nights out; prescriptions to pick up; phone calls to make (and return); plus all the day-to-day, run-of-the-mill stuff – drop-offs, pick-ups, lunchboxes, dinners, bath times, loads of washing. You had to get through it all, just to keep things ticking along. And I know I wasn't the only one who was feeling this way. I'm certain most of us feel this way at some point or other. But it's like you're trying hard to remember everything you need to do, but fail miserably on all counts.

That week I'd had a bit of a wobble about Oscar. The kind of wobble when you start questioning if you're doing enough for him, or if you could do more? I think every mum feels like they could spend more time with all their children, whether they have additional needs or not, but with the DS, that guilt rears its ugly head probably a little more frequently – much like the ugly head of my cold sore. Oscar had been unsettled, though, and not himself; sometimes I really wished he could just tell me what was up.

So, you remember Christmas 2016, when I talked about Oscar playing the part of a shepherd in his school nativity play and how he'd absolutely nailed it? [Insert smug face here.]

Ummmmmm, well, fast forward a whole year. To THIS particular year, Christmas 2017. When Oscar was given the part of one of the soldiers in the nativity. Well, this time, he was not having any of it.

In Oscar's defence, the previous year's play had been performed in the comfort of the village church. This year's was out on the school playground, meaning they were braving the elements and on the day of the 'show', it was pissing it down with rain. And it was cold, too. Mostly, he refused to stand up, even though the ground must have been cold and wet. And when he saw me in the audience, he got teary and spent the best part of the rest of the show standing with me, watching the rest of the school perform, a single tear rolling down his cheek because he really wasn't up for it AT ALL.

Once he'd gone back into class, the school were amazing and rang me straight afterwards to say he was fine. They said that he'd been brilliant at his soldier dance in rehearsals and very much a part of it all, but unfortunately, on the day, he just hadn't wanted to join in. I did, however, come away, having pinpointed two life lessons:

1. Oscar will always decide if he wants to do something. If he's not feeling it, it's not happening.
    and
2. NEVER be a Smug Mum, because no one likes you and you'll look like a nob when your kid doesn't do as well.

Oz had been poorly leading up to Christmas, which I now realise might have been why he was avoiding the nativity play. Whilst some children who are poorly might just have a little lie-down on the sofa, Oz goes the opposite way. He bounces off the walls. So much so that my calm, laid-back, chilled dude of a child turns into someone who is generally cross with life, and no amount of persuasion or reasoning seems to help. The school nativity that he'd basically refused outright to be a part of on the day had really knocked me for six. He'd taken part the previous year, so why hadn't he done so this time? It felt like a step backwards.

I'd also got into a bit of a flap about his speech. I mean, sure, he had a few high-frequency words that he'd chuck in here and there, but for the most part, at five-and-a-half years old, he was still pretty much non-verbal. Was it that he couldn't form the sounds? Was it that he was too scared to get it wrong because, occasionally, random, really hard words would pop out, like the time he said 'ambulance', but then it was never repeated? Or was it that this was simply it for him? That this, the handful of words he'd nailed, were the only words he'd ever say? There were moments, especially when I felt Oscar was having a hard time, or perhaps I was feeling low, that I really questioned Oscar's development, and if we were doing everything we could for him. I hated comparisons because I knew it was wasted energy, but I couldn't help comparing him with other children his age who were talking, reading and writing by now. He couldn't do any of this. And when, as a mother, you're having those moments, it's easy to go down a slippery slope, wondering if we were failing him, if we were truly doing enough to help him to be the best he could be. I'm hoping that one day I'll give myself a break and realise that we've all been doing the very best we can all along.

Christmas came and went, Oscar was well again and, with the new year, the kids were back to school and preschool. Don't get me wrong, I had loved having them home and it had been great to do fun school holiday stuff, but, truthfully, I still found it tough looking after three little ones. I remember around this time talking to a friend about my concerns that I hadn't been doing enough for Oscar to help him to learn. He had a profile online, where people were invested in his development and how he was getting on and I think, as a result, I felt pressure to show him in the best possible light, even though there were periods when it felt as though his development had come to a standstill. But it wasn't until I was talking to my friend, that something she said felt like a light-bulb moment for me. I'd said that in sharing Oscar's life online when we weren't having such a great time as far as behaviour and development were concerned, I felt pressure to remain positive and upbeat because others perceived Oscar's to be a success story, with regard to DS. My friend's response was, 'Oscar isn't a poster boy for Down syndrome. All our kids are different.' (She has a child with DS, too.)

And there it was.

She was so right.

I think I sometimes got too wrapped up in where I thought he should be and what he should be doing by a certain point. I knew it was ridiculous to compare him with other children his age who had DS, but sometimes I'd find myself doing so. When his little friend at the Christmas party of the charity we belong to called over to me saying, 'Sarah, come and sit next to me,' whilst I felt so chuffed that she was now able to say this amazing sentence, I also felt sad because I knew Oscar couldn't do the same. And for a while, I let moments like that overshadow everything Oscar was doing and how well he was getting on.

Perhaps having the blog and social media page added to that problem. I know that if I had been following myself, with a child younger than Oscar, I would have wanted to hear stories of hope, for the blog to show me how well Oscar was getting on. I would also want the posts to dispel a few myths about Down syndrome along the way. I knew I was guilty of getting too wrapped up in Oscar's development; it was time for me to stop thinking of him as a poster boy for Down syndrome. He was Oscar.

* * * *

Marriage is tough. I know I won't be the first or last to say it, but sometimes it really is. I don't often talk about Chris and my relationship publicly because I guess, despite being a self-confessed over-sharer, there are some things I feel should remain private. But Chris and our relationship are an integral part of our story. After the most depressingly wet and dismal weekend, having only been able to get out of the house briefly due to it being a wash-out, our relationship, it's fair to say, had been tested. I'm not sure if it's having had Oscar or, perhaps more significantly, having had three kids in close succession, but our children are the most incredible three things ever to have happened to us, it felt this particular weekend as if it had nearly broken us.

It was 4.55 a.m., I'd jumped into Oscar's bed when I'd heard him getting up and persuaded him to stay put. I'd put on *Gigglebiz* on the telly, silently willing him to stay quiet so that he didn't wake the other two. Life used to be a lot simpler when it was just Chris and me, but since having children, I think we've become less tolerant of one another. We bicker. Never about anything of substance. Always about the most insignificant, ridiculous things. The shouty-type whispers (so the kids don't hear), muttering under our breath, when undoubtedly you say stuff to each other that you'd never dream of saying to your mate or a family member because, well, you live and breathe one another, so it's somehow got to the point that it feels like you can. I think the nub of the problem is the push-pull in the relationship. Who's the most tired? Who's under the most pressure or is the most stressed? And it becomes about who trumps whom, I guess. I work hard to provide for us as a family, Chris says. But I stay home, cook, clean and care for the kids, work AND hold my shit together, I reply. All of this is internal, of course. Neither of us at this stage had ever actually said any of that out loud, but I'm certain it's what we were both thinking.

We'd met up with some friends who'd just been away as they were celebrating thirty years of marriage. They had two grown-up children and, from the outside looking in, seemed to be very much in love. In a quiet moment, I got talking to the wife and I blurted out something about marriage being hard and what was their secret. Her response, however, stopped me in my tracks when she responded that, for them, it hadn't been hard at all. That, if anything, it had been easy.

Had she just forgotten what it was like to have small children? Was their relationship so solid that the introduction of three or, in her case two, smalls hadn't come close to breaking them? Were Chris and I different to most? Her words really stayed with me.

The truth is, this was us. Warts and all. It wasn't plain sailing; there'd been ripples on the sea. Sometimes damn big waves. I think sometimes we forgot to be kind to one another, to see how hard the other was working. Sometimes life gets in the way.

This weekend, however, we'd made it outside briefly. The kids had been HARD WORK, it was pouring with rain and, as we were walking back to the car, I had a bit of a moment. It was literally chucking it down, the kids had had enough and Oscar and Alfie had both retreated to the buggy. Chris was pushing them, neither of them were strapped in and, as we approached the traffic lights to cross a very busy main road, we stood and waited. Chris and I knew that Alfie wouldn't have even thought about getting out of the buggy and crossing until he saw the green man or heard the signal, but Oz, although it was unlikely that he would, still wasn't at the stage where we could completely trust him not to. And as we stood there in silence, I saw that Chris had positioned himself to the side of the buggy on which Oscar was sitting, ready to stop him running across the road if he needed to. As it happened, Oscar didn't move a muscle, but Chris being there, at Oscar's side, ready to save him if needed, reminded me that we've so got this. This parenthood lark, I mean.

After we'd crossed the road, I told Chris I'd noticed what he'd done, how without having to say a word, we'd been on the same page. He'd had it covered. Being a parent is tough. But being married is sometimes tougher. We aren't perfect. I know we've never been that. But sometimes, in moments like that, it's the kids who are the glue that hold us together. We needed to give each other a break, we needed to be nicer to one another, but we also needed to remember how all of this had started sometimes. With just us.

Over the years, things have got easier. The children have grown older and don't need us in the same way they once did. I think what's helped our relationship, too, is me finding a new career and a renewed sense of direction, as one thing I was passionate about after having Oscar was that I didn't want to be known only as Oscar's mum. Sure, Oscar and the care he requires play a big part in my day-to-day life, but somewhere along the way, when the kids were small, I felt like I'd lost *me* for a while, and I'd known that for the sake of our kids and our marriage, I had to find Sarah again.

Blog Comments

'A colleague of my husband, a Professor of Astrophysics, who happened to be from Greece, with degrees from both Thessaloniki and Cambridge(!), told us of a "cure" she'd read about which was hanging my child upside down so that oxygen could flood her brain as people with Down syndrome were lacking.'

Sarah Illingworth

'From my own mother, while poring over the baby a week after he'd been born (it took her THAT long to visit us in hospital) – "He doesn't look too bad." And, then she offered how she felt about Kyle having DS, "I was very disappointed." Suffice it to say, we don't see her any more!'

Anon

'A GP once asked me if I took drugs or drank alcohol while I was pregnant because it was unusual for someone of my age (I was twenty-nine) to have a baby with DS.'

Sarah Saunders

10

'She Shouldn't Have to Feel Grateful'

I knew that other children Oscar's age had the opportunity to attend various holiday clubs, football camps, play schemes and so on, which I knew Oscar would love, but I knew that he wasn't ready for those just yet. I was keen for Oscar to be able to access something like this. Also, I had always been mindful that in a mainstream setting like that the ratio of adults to kids is likely to be lower and asking someone to be Oscar's 1:1 – when there weren't necessarily the resources – would have been a big ask. I also knew that these clubs weren't technically allowed to turn him down under the discrimination act, but I still had my reservations about him going, being so young still and being as unpredictable as he was then. He'd have needed a 1:1 and if there weren't enough staff to cover that, I would have felt too cautious about leaving him.

Challengers is a scheme that offers play and leisure opportunities for disabled children in Surrey, Hampshire, and beyond. Each day during the holidays, they set up different areas for the kids to play in. They have a soft-play area, computers, the most incredible outside space for accessible bikes, trikes, go-karts, ball games, sand and water play, the largest children's play structure you've ever seen, that Oscar gets to climb on, slide down and run around in. There is also a quiet space for downtime.

In 2015, it was found that 86 per cent of disabled children didn't have access to regular play or leisure activities, I imagine primarily due to that lack of funding. So that's why Challengers was just brilliant for Oscar. It is a registered charity and, although we paid for Oscar to attend, it was heavily subsidised. Challengers still relies to a large extent on donations and fundraising to keep the scheme running.

When Oscar is at Challengers, he doesn't have a 1:1 as they, and we, feel he can cope well in that environment. The play scheme is heavily staffed and there's no way he could get up to too much mischief, so I have always felt confident that he is more than looked after there.

I love that it gives him some independence and a chance to have fun, but it also gives me the extra time to spend with Alfie and Flo, something parents of a child with 'needs' often feel a huge amount of guilt about: not spending enough time with the siblings, I mean.

For February half-term I'd signed Oz up for a session at Challengers. He was thrilled to be going and always very excited when we drove up. And I realised, while he was there, just how much more relaxed I felt without him around, having just the other two to look after. I hope that doesn't make me sound too awful, admitting that out loud, but it was very much my reality. It's not to say he was a nightmare or that it hasn't got a bit easier since he's grown older because he's not, and it has, but when he was around, certainly back then, I always had to be one step ahead of him, pre-empting what he'd do next. When we were out and about, I could never really afford to let my guard down, just in case, and even in the house, although he couldn't do too much damage, I'd always be listening out for what he was up to. Examples in February half-term week were: going into the playroom that had just been decorated, getting the roller, which still had paint on it, and painting our newly painted wall in another room; grabbing the pillows and duvet off our bed and throwing it all down the stairs; emptying all the recycling bins all over the kitchen floor; and climbing onto the kitchen worktop, all the while dancing to the *Gigglebiz* theme tune. It was affirmative: this kid kept me on my toes. So, for the three hours that morning, while he was having a brilliant time at Challengers, I got the chance to concentrate on Alfie and Flo, before the madness recommenced that afternoon. Families like mine benefit so greatly from organisations like this one. I know that we, for one, are truly grateful for the opportunities he has because of them, and I feel passionate about them continuing because they can be a lifeline for so, so many.

Jumping ahead to a little later that year, however, I did decide to approach a local mainstream holiday club, to explore the possibility of Oscar joining them during the holidays. There was one that came highly recommended to us, so they were my first port of call. You see, Oz loves sports. He'll often sit – well, usually stand – next to the TV when Chris is watching the rugby, get really into it in all the right places and clap and cheer when it all goes Chris's team's way. When the big kids in the park are having a kick-about with a football, given half a chance, Oscar would be the first one to try to get involved. So, I guess when I contacted them, I thought it'd be lovely if, like some of his peers, Oz had the opportunity to attend too. And all the while, I wasn't denying the fact that he would need to be supported while he was there, but I knew that with that support he'd have the best time.

I'd written to the local organisation to ask how they'd feel about Oscar attending. I wrote how I understood that it would cost them more money to provide a 1:1 for him, but that if they didn't have the extra provision in place, we'd be happy to cover the cost. I asked if they knew of a young student who might want some experience working with a child like Oscar. I'd written a bit about what sort of support he'd need, which ultimately boiled down to keeping him on task and making sure he didn't wander off, basically keeping him safe. I'd also said that although Oscar had made some progress with his toileting, he would still need help with this.

This was the response I received:

Hi Sarah

Thank you for your email. We would be happy to help and provide you with 1:1 support if you were to pay extra.

However, the only issue we have is the toileting. As we are sports coaches, we are not allowed to help with that element.

Perhaps you could come back to me when he is able to go alone?

Many thanks

It felt like a sucker punch. I mean, to a point, I got it. I understood about safeguarding as far as taking him to the toilet or changing a pull-up was concerned. I understood they were a business and that having a child like Oscar would be extra work for them, but I'm not sure, in all my years, I had ever received an email that felt like more of a blow to the stomach than this one had been.

It was a few lines. It felt like they weren't even open to discussion and finding a solution and that hurt. I could have replied with a long-winded response about inclusion, about how their website very clearly states that they want to provide for 'all' children and thrown in the disability discrimination act about how, in theory, they should be making 'reasonable adjustments'. I'm sure I would have got what I'd wanted in the end, had I really pushed, but the truth was, if an organisation like this one didn't want to help, if it didn't want to find a way around a problem but would rather simply give up at the first hurdle, I wasn't sure it was the right place for Oscar anyway. Some days, as a mum, you feel like you can move mountains. Others? You just feel sad for your little boy that things aren't just that little bit easier for him.

Fast forward another three years and just a few short months ago, a friend of mine who runs a similar club told me they'd had an email from a mum of a child who happens to have DS. She'd asked if she could pay for a 1:1 so that they could be included, and my friend told me they'd thought of Oscar straight away. They also told me that they'd gone straight back to this mum and said that they'd be THRILLED to have this child and that, although it would take some planning, it was essentially a YES!

We discussed afterwards how the mother had been so grateful to my friend and how my friend had found this tough, saying, 'She shouldn't have to feel grateful, Sarah.

This child should be offered the same opportunities as the next.'

And then I felt emotional, because I knew my friend understood – and I loved them for that – but also because I understood too well those feelings of gratitude myself.

I'm probably going to get some stick for this because often I feel the consensus among parents of children with SEN, is 'Why shouldn't they be included?' but here's the thing, genuinely? I'm grateful when someone suggests a play date with Oscar. In the same way I'm grateful when he's invited to a birthday party of a classmate from his old school. I'm grateful when someone tells me their child loves mine and I know I'd be super-grateful if someone were to give him a place at their club, despite it being undeniably harder work to have him there. And the reason I'm grateful is because none of the above is a given for us. He's not always invited, or always accepted, or always loved. And no matter how much we try to change the narrative, 'acceptance' will always be a hurdle for him.

Unless you have first-hand experience, I don't expect you to get it, but I just think it's so important if someone runs a club, class, group or team that if they have the chance to give a child like Oz the opportunity to give it a go, they should never underestimate how much that 'YES' means.

Walking home from school one afternoon, from his second year in reception, Oscar stopped in his tracks, took his backpack off and started to open it. He'd obviously remembered there was something in there that he wanted to show me and he pulled out a handwritten envelope with his name on the front. We waited until we got home and opened it together. It read:

Dear Oscar,

You're funny and you make me laugh

Love *****

xxxxxxxxx

The note was from a little girl in Oscar's class, who, when I messaged her mum to tell her how chuffed he'd been when I'd read it out, said that her daughter calls him her boyfriend and that she'd been insistent that she write to him. As a mum of a child with additional needs, there are moments from time to time when you wonder if you've done the right thing. You worry that the gap between your child and their mainstream peers is too wide. I worried less about this gap academically speaking in that if he was making progress and feeling like he was achieving, to my mind that was enough. But the social side of things had always been a big worry of mine. Did the other kids want to play with him? Was he included? Did he have friends? But then there were the moments like this one, when I paused, just for a second, and remembered exactly why a mainstream school was the best place for Oscar at that point.

We found out that evening that Alfie would be joining Oscar at the school in September. We had assumed that he'd get in based on the sibling rule, but I will admit to having had a minor panic, wondering if I'd filled the form in correctly. I loved the fact that, come September, they'd be at the school together, to look out for one another from time to time. I didn't know for how long. At that stage, Oz might have gone all the way through his education in a mainstream school or he might only have managed mainstream for a short while. Either way, knowing that the two boys would be with each other later that year and knowing that Oz had got a little girlfriend there, well, that made me smile, just as much as he had been smiling that evening.

* * * *

In January the previous year, Oscar had had surgery to remove the cholesteatoma that had been found growing in his left ear during a routine grommet insertion. After another procedure at the end of the same year to check it hadn't grown back, whilst it had not returned in *that* ear, another had been found growing in his other ear. The first surgery to remove the cholesteatoma from his right ear lasted five-and-a-half hours – the longest wait ever – and whilst it wasn't as extensive a growth as the previous one, his surgeon said it had grown considerably, so this operation took just as long. Oscar had more of a wait to go down to theatre, as his surgery didn't start until 2 p.m. This meant that we had more time to keep him occupied beforehand and the longer wait, combined with the fact that he hadn't eaten or drunk anything for hours, meant that he was really upset by the time he went to sleep. Chris was with us at the hospital, but as he really doesn't like the bit where they give Oscar his general anaesthetic, I opted to be with him for this. Normally, I'm tough and hold it together, but seeing him so distressed and having to literally hold him to me with all my strength, I lost it this time. It was so heart-breaking.

They managed to remove all of the cholesteatoma, which thankfully hadn't caused too much damage. His ear was then packed with cotton while it healed. They'd need to take out the packing, under general anaesthetic again, in three weeks' time, but because they had gone in behind the ear through his skull again, he had a cut from just behind the top of the ear down to the bottom. We'd been told he needed ten days, two weeks, off school to allow the scar to heal. He was to be discharged the following day, so Chris stayed in with him overnight. It had been a long day, but a successful one, and I felt relieved it was all over again, for a while at least.

* * * *

A teeny-tiny step in gentle education: in spring 2018, I gave a talk to a group of student midwives at Anglia Ruskin University, in Chelmsford. What I didn't know was that sitting in that lecture theatre listening to me was a representative from the Royal College of Midwives, who came over to speak to me afterwards. We exchanged contact details and have been in touch again more recently. As a result, the *Don't Be Sorry* website and social media channels are now officially listed in the resources section of the module called 'Delivering unexpected news'. This means that any student midwife currently in training will have access to my blog page, which will hopefully give them an insight into not only the importance of the language they use, but also how they approach and handle 'new' mothers, when they are finding out that their little one has DS. It means, too, that they can point the new mums in our direction if they feel they might need support. A small step, but a huge one for the DS community.

* * * *

113

Oscar was turning six in July and occasionally I would be asked if Alfie and Flo knew that he had Down syndrome. Up until this point, it wasn't something we'd ever discussed with them as I genuinely don't think it had occurred to either of them that Oscar was any 'different' to anyone else. However, one day, a friend of Alfie's came over, someone who hadn't spent much time with Oscar before, and while Oscar, Alfie, Flo and this little girl played so well together, over tea she asked me straight out, 'How come Oscar can't talk? I thought you said he was five?' As Oscar's grown older, I have noticed more and more that children around his age are picking up on the fact that he may be a little different from them. Obviously, there are going to be some kids who are more perceptive about these things than others, but Alfie and Flo at this point hadn't really said too much. They'd never asked why he sometimes behaved the way he did, why he was the one I held onto when we were all walking down a busy street, or even why I was STILL changing his pull-up. To them, he was just Oscar. One thing I did pick up on, though, was Alfie's ability at just four years old (and seventeen months his big brother's junior) to look out for Oz. Whether it be in the playground, the park, soft play. . . he always had his back.

It's known in our family that, over the years, Alfie's had a bit of bad press. I'm not going to lie, out of the three of them, he was probably the one who challenged me the most with his behaviour and perhaps the one I've moaned about the most, but as he's grown older, he hasn't been doing so badly. Just the other day, on our way home from preschool, Flo chirped up from the back of the car that one of the other little boys there had supposedly hit her earlier that day. Anyone who's ever spent more than two minutes around my children will know that none of them is an angel and my immediate thought was that she had probably done something to provoke this. So I asked her why he'd hit her and, before she'd even had a chance to answer, Alfie jumped in with, 'Yes, he did hit her, but don't wowwy, I hit him back and then I sat on him.'

Now of course I explained to him that, even though it was lovely that he'd stuck up for his little sister, violence isn't the right way to respond to violence and that it's never acceptable to hit others. I'm pretty sure he understood, but there was also a small part of me that wanted to tell him that I thought he was ace. That I LOVED that he'd stuck up for Flo and that, secretly, although it's not the 'done thing' to admit it out loud, I felt proud that he'd do that for her. When I had Oscar and then subsequently went on to have Alfie and Flo, people told me that they'd have a bond, but I never fully got it. In much the same way that Alfie sees Flo as his sister, I love that he also just sees Oscar as Oscar. I know that he'll have further questions as time goes by and, when he does, we'll be ready for them, but for now, he sees Oscar for the brother that he is. Nothing more, nothing less.

Blog Comments

'My sister Jacqueline is five years older than me and has DS. She will be fifty-two this year and leads a very full and active life. Following my dad's passing last year, she went to live with my sister and brother-in-law and soon realised that she would be treated no differently to anyone else. She contributes to the household and takes a turn of chores etc., things that my dad had always done for her, and probably didn't need to. She makes us laugh every day and is always there with a smile and a squeezy hug and will sign, "I love you". Best sibling ever in my opinion.'

@chrissyghirl

'We have three children: our daughter is eight and our twin boys are five. One twin has DS. They all love each other dearly. The twins started mainstream school together in September, the same school our daughter attends. Just after half-term, our daughter asked if she could speak to the whole school about Henry, because they treat him like a baby. She wrote an assembly which basically said, "He may be small, but he is mighty, and he may not get things at the same time as everyone else, but he will get there with our support." I was so proud of her.'

Tammy Fitzjohn

'Betsy is the youngest of three girls: Rose (9), Ruby (7) and Betsy (2). They treat her very typically for the most part, they understand she has DS and it's no big deal to them.

Rose asked me a little while ago why did I cry so much when I was pregnant with Betsy, and I knew I needed to be honest, so I told her I was frightened because Betsy would have DS. Rose looked me straight in the eye, let out a belly roar of laughter and said, "Oh, Mummy, what a silly billy," and I began to laugh too and said, "What a silly billy," and I really meant it. They are fiercely protective and say her DS is her superpower. God help anyone who disagrees.'

Kelly Marshall

11

'Small Steps Every Day'

'Your story is unique and so, so different
and not worthy of comparison'
Unknown

When Oscar was a baby and a toddler, I would forever find myself comparing him with his peers. And when I say peers, I don't mean other children who happened to have Down syndrome, I mean those 'typically developing' children whom we'd meet in his nursery, at our local playgroup or in the park. I would find myself thinking, 'Well, that's good because Oscar can keep up with them in most areas,' and I guess that somehow, that made things easier.

But as he'd grown older and I suppose, to an extent, that gap had widened, I didn't do it any more. What I remained guilty of was occasionally comparing his development to that of his peers who have DS. Another little boy might have been reading well and able to say the sentences out loud, whereas Oscar might have been able only to recognise some words and, even if he could have read it all, he wouldn't have been able to say the words out loud.

Someone else might have been writing in full sentences whereas we were happy if Oscar had managed to write the first letter of his name.

So, when Oscar attended one of his mainstream peer's birthday parties, along with most of his class, I guess I just assumed that Oscar wouldn't be able to keep up. But, as the party went on, I realised he wasn't struggling at all. In fact, he was holding his own, behaving just like all his mainstream peers and was very much part of the group. Other children spoke to him, laughed along with him, played with him, helped him if he needed it. And before, where I would have been just a few steps behind him, just in case he did something he shouldn't, this time I stood back and watched. And do you know what? Not for one single second of that party did he let himself down once.

It was one of those times I realised not only how far he'd come, but also how important it was for him then to be around other kids his age. Not because he was keeping up academically – some days that side of things felt so ridiculously slow that I wondered if he was ever going to get there – but because it reminded me what a waste of time and energy it was to compare him with any other child, whether they had DS or not. Watching him at that party I saw just how important the social side of things was for him, and he was doing brilliantly.

There was one little girl at the party who spent a bit more time with him. I'd never seen the interaction between the two of them before because obviously I wasn't in the classroom with them at school. So, on the way out, as we were saying goodbye, I turned to the mother of this little girl and said, 'She's really great with him, you know?'

And her reply, as if it was the most natural, most obvious thing in the world, was, 'She loves him.'

Sometimes you've just got to take a step back and have a little faith – that everything is going to be okay.

As the academic year ended, Oscar took part in his annual school sports day again. I'm not sure he mastered every skill, e.g. I'm pretty sure the beanbag was supposed to be balanced on top of the tennis racket, rather than being pinned against it, and that technically he was supposed to have weaved in and out of the coloured markers on the floor instead of smiling for the camera, looking at me and living his best life. If I remember correctly, I'm also pretty sure he came in last in both the running and the obstacle races, and that he knocked down the bar on the high jump EVERY SINGLE TIME. But for every ball he threw and caught, every goal he scored, every frisbee he tossed, every hula hoop he spun and with every whack of the hockey stick, the expression on his face was priceless. He loved every second of it. It's not the winning, it's the taking part that counts, they say. Never a truer word has been said.

* * * *

Every Monday, Oscar had speech therapy, when his therapist would visit him at school and, at the beginning of the term, would set him ongoing targets. One of the targets set for this particular term was for Oscar to able to go up to a peer in his class and initiate play. Knowing how highly motivated Oscar was to play with the other children, as a reward at the end of his SALT (speech and language therapy) sessions, he got to choose a friend he'd like to play with (from a little book they'd made of everyone's names and faces), go up to them in the classroom and try to say, 'Come and play.' He'd known the signs, had attempted to say the words each week and he'd been so pleased that he was now able to do this.

After successfully choosing a friend to play with and them finishing their game together, it was then time for that child to go back to the class, so Oscar could finish up his session before joining them. But one day Oscar, apparently, as clear as day, turned to his friend and said, 'Thank you, bye,' without prompting from any adult. He simply said it, just like that. Speech had been Oscar's biggest hurdle. He would very occasionally pull out the odd new word, but progress up until this stage had been super-slow. So, you can imagine how delighted we were when I opened his communication book that afternoon and read, 'Small steps every day'.

It was my fortieth birthday that particular year. I remembered when I was in my twenties, thinking that forty seemed so far off. The truth was, now that I was there, it hadn't been that far off at all. I'm not altogether sure where I thought I'd be at this stage of life because I don't think when I was in my twenties I thought much past my career, friendship groups, boys and the latest 'on trend' outfit from Topshop. I think, if I really analyse it, I was kind of wrapped up in the here and now and wasn't thinking much past the next week. I'd always assumed I'd get married, have kids and it would all work out, but having lived a bit more of life now, I realise that nothing is a certainty and people don't always get the happy ending they imagined they would.

Ten years earlier, on my thirtieth birthday, Chris, whom I'd never met before, had walked up to me in a bar, handed me a large glass of white wine and said, 'I'm Chris. Happy Birthday!' He'd tagged along to my party as the guest of my now brother-in-law and at the time, to be honest, apart from liking his muscles – shallow, I know – and thinking he seemed like a nice enough guy, I didn't think much more than that. Fast forward a few months, and I had a friend request from him on Facebook and an invitation to see Elton John in concert at the O2 (I mean, a man who loves Elton John – match made in heaven or what?) Well, the rest is history. If someone had told me ten years ago, however, that in ten years' time I would have given up my career as a dancer because, in the end, after eight years of doing it, I just fell out of love with it, I don't think I would have believed them. That was all I'd ever wanted, you see. If they'd said that my work now would involve writing, social media influencing and public speaking, again, I wouldn't have believed them, and if they'd said that I'd be married to 'Muscles' from the bar, that we'd have three kids so ridiculously close in age that I'd essentially been pregnant for most of 2012 through to the summer of 2015 and that one of those kids would have Down syndrome – if someone had told me all of that – well, I think I'd have laughed in their face. I mean, that wasn't the way it was supposed to go, right?

Although at the time I'd thought Oscar's diagnosis was the worst news imaginable and I'd spent the first few months worrying that I didn't have the first clue how to parent, let alone a kid with 'needs', and although I wasn't the slightest bit like the type of mother I'd thought I'd be, I'd also have laughed if they'd told me that I'd not done that badly.

Life wasn't perfect. I'd learnt that over my forty years. I didn't get enough sleep, yet I stayed up late watching *Love Island* every night. When I got cross about somebody calling me out on something, it was usually because I knew there was an element of truth in what they were saying, and I was embarrassed that they'd got the measure of me. I wasn't strict enough with my kids because, mostly, I was just trying to get through each day, and I sometimes couldn't be arsed with the fight. I'd lost touch with a handful of lovely, long-term friends that I wished I hadn't. Equally, when new people walked into my life, I'd sometimes be really rubbish at making the effort with them because that had required too much energy, too. I had vowed at the start of that year that by my fortieth birthday I'd be at least two stone lighter. Had I done it? Had I bo*****s. I tried and failed with healthy eating almost every Monday. Life WASN'T perfect, but I realise now, it probably wasn't for anyone I knew. So, heading into my fortieth year, as a surprise, Muscles had booked us a night away in Amsterdam. I had no idea where we were going until I got to the departure lounge. As we headed onto the plane, he'd handed me a piece of paper and written on it was the poem, 'Welcome to Holland' by Emily Pearl Kingsley, which I'd been sent when I'd been in hospital with Oscar, having just given birth to him. Now, lots of people have mixed feelings about the poem but I know that in those early few days after having given birth to Oscar, that poem truly helped me. It talks about how you're going on a trip and you think you're headed to Italy, only there's been a change of plan and you've now landed in Holland. You hadn't wanted to go to Holland though, as you didn't think it was anywhere near as amazing as Italy. Italy was fast-paced and flash. Holland was a lot slower, and full of clogs. But do you know what? Now that I've seen Holland first-hand and spent some time there, I was almost certain it didn't get any better than that. Chris and I had a whirlwind trip to Amsterdam. My mum and dad looked after the kids and

Chris and I got some time together to reconnect. Having young kids was hard, but having a child like Oscar, with the extra challenges (mostly lack of sleep) took its toll from time to time, and we'd needed some time for just the two of us.

* * * *

Every single audiology appointment over the past six years had shown that Oscar has, depending on the day, mild to moderate hearing loss. When he was younger, he'd worn a BAHA hearing band for a while, but having had a break from that to see how he got on without it, both his audiologist and his ENT consultant had recently discussed reintroducing a hearing aid. Whether it was the glue ear to blame or the cholesteatoma, either way, something was impacting on his hearing and it wasn't improving. So, you can imagine how pleased we were to find out at his next appointment that, despite having congestion in both ears – we thought because he'd had a nasty cold the previous month and it was taking a while to clear – that he'd absolutely smashed his test. He sat beautifully throughout, followed instructions perfectly and completed each stage of the hearing test. He didn't do his usual 'I'm going to pretend I'm not listening to you because I'm so over putting these ridiculous little men in a boat every time I hear a noise'; instead, he'd stayed completely focused and on task. And right at the very end of the test, they said that his hearing was now within 'normal' range in both ears!!! Up until then, we had literally NEVER had a clear test. EVER!

* * * *

For the past three years, Oscar and I, with our friends Karen and her little boy Lance, have made the 264-mile round trip to the School of Optometry and Vision Sciences at the University of Cardiff. You see, every year, the boys have an appointment with an amazing lady who specialises in testing the eyesight of young people who happen to have Down syndrome and who, for the past twenty years or so, has been running a study of visual development in others just like Lance and Oscar. Having had his eyes tested multiple times from a very early age, Lance was compliant in his test every single time. Whereas with Oscar, who freaked out at most appointments with professionals (because, I figure, having had numerous operations and procedures by now, he looks at a person coming towards him and wonders what's about to happen next), it had always been notoriously difficult to get the results required.

However, this time we arrived, it was suggested that Lance and Oscar went in together because then Oscar could watch Lance and see that, actually, there wasn't anything to worry about. My immediate thought was that we couldn't possibly do that as I didn't want us putting Lance off, especially if Oscar freaked out and caused mass hysteria – it has been known. But remembering that Oscar really loved to get things right and that he often did copy other children's behaviour, I quickly decided that we could only give it a go.

Lance had gone first and Oscar, who was sitting some distance away from what was happening, watched intently. From time to time, having tested Lance on something, the optometrist would then turn to Oscar and do the same. The boys took it in turns to name all the objects on the cards, up close and then from a distance. Lance was now managing to name all the objects which he hadn't quite had the speech to do the previous year. Oz, too, showed that he knew all the signs for the objects and he also tried his best to say some of the words. It had been such a lovely moment to watch and showed again the progress our kids can make. The trip to Wales was a huge success, in that this year was the first time Oscar had co-operated, remained calm and they'd been able to get a detailed enough report to know that his eyesight was good for now.

Around this time, Seeability, the charity which works to ensure that all young people who have additional needs are being tested by an optometrist who has a full understanding of what their needs might be, got in touch with me. Their take on things is that children like Oscar may be more apprehensive at first. They may take more time to grasp what's required of them and they may not have the concentration skills. For a lot of children with additional needs, anything out of the ordinary, like someone trying to look into the depths of their eyes, may be a traumatic ordeal if performed by someone who doesn't know the right approach to take. So Seeability were trying to ensure that properly trained people were in these positions.

As things stood back then, if you were in a mainstream school you would be offered an eye test in reception. However, if you'd been in a SEN setting, eye tests weren't being offered at all. That meant that thousands of children with learning disabilities were missing out on crucial eye care, despite being twenty-eight times more likely to have a sight problem. Just insane.

We were fortunate enough to be able to travel to Cardiff to see a specialist in this field, whose attitude was that one size didn't always fit all. She was patient and was adaptable to each individual child's needs. And I couldn't help thinking how amazing it would be if under every local service there was someone trained up like her?

* * * *

It was Oscar's final day of reception, a class he'd been in for the past two years. All the emotions of the last day of term snuck up on me in a big way that day and I was very emotional. It was not only Oscar's last day in reception, but also Alfie's final day in preschool before he moved up to big school.

Alfie had been at his preschool for the previous two years and had formed a lovely bond with his key person, whom he'd always called 'My Sally'. So, when HIS Sally started getting teary that morning, it set me off. I genuinely had no idea that I would feel so sad. The other thing that set me off was that in all the time Oscar had been at school, he'd always had the same morning TA for the two years he'd been in reception. She'd been with him from the very start, but sadly, for us, because he was moving up to Year One, the school felt that come September it would be in Oscar's best interests for him to work with a different 1:1 in her place. I don't think I'm alone in saying this, but when you get it right, there's something special about the bond between a child and their TA. I guess it's because they're spending so much of their time with one another. But, in short, I couldn't fault her if I tried. And although I had every confidence in the school with the choices they made for Oscar, it felt like we were starting all over again with the anxiety and worry, wondering if it would all work out.

So here we were, the summer holidays had arrived, our snack cupboards were filled, our iPads charged, and our gin cupboards well and truly stocked.

Blog Comments

'Leo's first speech and language therapist was a wonderful American lady. She was the person who explained to us that while typically developing children may pick up a new skill within four or five attempts, a child with additional needs may take up to 100 exposures – she gave us so much hope.'

Tessa Cliff Reid

'We had a wonderful physio for twelve years. She used to pop in and check on us when she wasn't even booked to see us, taught me how to do different exercises/moves with my girls, came to appointments with us and just always listened to me and any worries I had. I don't think she realised how much she meant to me and my girls, but she was one of a kind.'

Luwan Paling

'I'll never forget Lisa, the NICU family liaison, who I saw for counselling sessions while struggling to deal with the challenges ahead. She'd previously been a NICU nurse so she just "got it" and she always made sure to make a fuss of my son and tell me how beautiful he was. That was important at a time when I wasn't yet quite able to see that myself, through the grief and fear.'

Sarah Waugh

'I was at a routine antenatal appointment about a month after finding out that Tills had DS. She asked me a question and I remember replying, "You do know my baby has Down syndrome?" What she said next changed so much for me. "I do know, and I just want to say, thank you. Thank you for being here, thank you for the beautiful baby you will have and thank you for letting us be able to care for you." When you're entering an unknown world, it meant so much to feel wanted.'

Abi Lethbridge

12

The Love Stuff Knocks You Sideways

*'We don't grow when things are easy,
we grow when we face challenges'*
Unknown

I'd been invited to Hayling Island beach with some friends,
and I'd been a bit dubious about going. That was mainly
because we were still in that place where subjecting myself
to sole parenting in any wide-open space, where all three
children were likely to go off in different directions, was
just something I would try desperately to avoid. If we were
to go somewhere like that, I'd always have another adult
with me – Chris, my parents, my sisters – just in case.
But this day, I'd decided that I couldn't keep saying no to
invitations and, as lovely as my family were about coming
along, I couldn't keep roping them in, so I'd braved it:
me, three kids, the beach, a WIDE-OPEN SPACE, where
they were all free to go wherever the hell they liked and a
shedload of water!

My friends – altogether we had fifteen children with
us – were on standby if I needed it, but I was conscious
that they all had their own children to keep tabs on too.

It didn't go unnoticed, however, that when needed, they had my back. One would watch Alfie in the water, while I followed Oz, who had decided he needed to go back to the picnic area we'd finished in over half an hour ago, to get his grapes. As I was clearing up Flo's sticky hands from an ice lolly, another friend hotfooted it after Oscar, who'd decided to walk into an unsuspecting lady's beach hut and take a seat on her stool. Thankfully she'd been lovely about it but the take-home for me that day was that I didn't once feel anxious or like I hadn't got control of the situation. The kids – that's mine and the other twelve of them – all genuinely behaved beautifully and, if anything, I had felt really relaxed. I loved that I'd got to paddle in the sea with them, bury our toy dinosaurs in the pebbles and watch them play with their friends. It was the kind of day I imagine I'll always remember.

I will just say as an aside, a top tip for any parent whose child is a runner, plonking yourself on a pebble-filled beach for the day basically meant that even if Oscar had wanted to run, he couldn't, because, let's face it, it ruddy well hurts when you try running on stones. I'd therefore call that mummy for the win!

* * * *

One day I was out shopping with the kids when a woman stopped us and said, 'I recognise you. . . I follow your blog.' It's always nice when someone stops me to say hi, but after chatting for a little while and having said our goodbyes, I couldn't help thinking about what she'd said. She'd said she'd been following us for a while as she had a thirty-three-year-old daughter called Becky [not her real name] who happens to have Down syndrome too. This lady was pushing her granddaughter in the trolley and, after a minute or so of talking together, I realised that her daughter Becky was with her in the shop and had gone off on her own to find a chocolate dessert she wanted. This lady told me that she had three daughters and that the little girl in the trolley was Becky's niece. She'd told me that Becky had a job and didn't live with her any more; she now lived independently. In the few minutes that I stood and chatted to her, I could tell she was a kind woman. Without my prompting, she told me that times have changed and that she knew Oscar would be okay because if he was anything like Becky, he'd lead a great life. I told her that there'd always been a niggling worry in the back of my mind about the future and that all I'd wanted was for him to be happy. Hopefully he'd get a job and live independently. 'That was the end goal,' I'd told her.

But she'd stopped me in my tracks when she very matter-of-factly said, 'Yes, I know what you mean, but I've always felt that I didn't have my children to send them away.'

It stopped me in my tracks because I guess I'd always imagined that your child being able to live independently was what everyone who has a child with Down syndrome wishes for. Most of us, I felt, would want that they could live independently. But she then went on to say that while it was great that Becky lived independently, she loved it when Becky came home. She said that when her other daughter's husband was away with work, she'd often come and stay with her, so why should it be any different with Becky. She wanted her to come home. She also told me that, sadly, about three years ago, her husband (Becky and her sisters' father) had passed away. There was a sadness in her eyes when she spoke of him. I automatically assumed that as her mum, this woman would be the one comforting and reassuring Becky after her dad's passing. I assumed that Becky would be the one needing her mum and while I'm sure this woman had been a huge strength to Becky when she'd needed it, the general feeling I got was that it was the other way round, that this woman probably needed Becky just as much. She went on to say that she and Becky went on holidays together. By the sounds of things, they'd also hang out on the weekends, but she was quick to say that she was still mindful that she wanted Becky to have her own life. I know sometimes people think that adults with DS are a burden on their families. As their typically developing peers grow up, find jobs, and move out of home, there's a general feeling that people with DS are going to get left behind. But as I thought about this family's dynamic, it made me smile thinking about how they were there for one another. As we said goodbye, Becky, having waited patiently for her mum and me to stop talking, turned to her and said, 'Sorry, Mum, I've looked for it, but I can't find that chocolate pudding anywhere.' I forget her exact words now, but her mum reassured her that she'd help her try to find it. The reply itself was insignificant, really. What I loved about it was it was one of the most normal, simplest of exchanges between a mother and daughter and left me feeling happy that they had each other. I came home and told Chris about meeting Becky and, as usual, as I waffled on, he appeared not really to be listening to me. (I do have a habit of going on.) But, right at the end, he came back with the same response he'd been making for the past six years when I've spoken about Oz being independent. He said, 'Listen, I'm happy if Oscar always lives with us. But I've told you, if/when we move, I'm going to build him a little house at the bottom of the garden, so he's always with us.'

* * * *

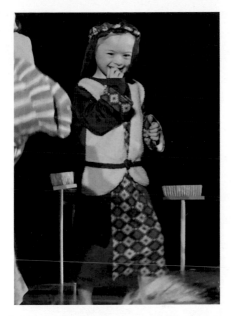

Oscar loving the limelight in his school nativity play.
(13 December 2018)

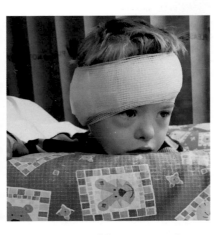

Mr Bump! Oscar following surgery for a
cholesteatoma in his ear.
(10 January 2019)

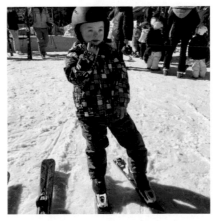

Oscar hits the slopes on his second skiing holiday.
(16 February 2019)

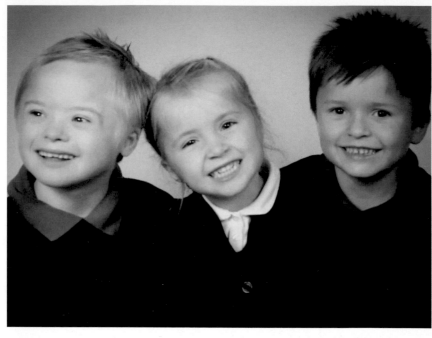

The first and last photo of Oscar, Flo and Alfie all at the same school together.
(10 December 2019)

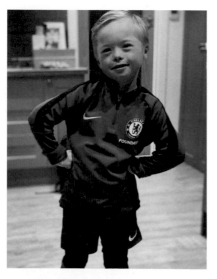

Oscar proudly wearing his football kit for the
Chelsea Football Foundation, which he loved.
(17 February 2020)

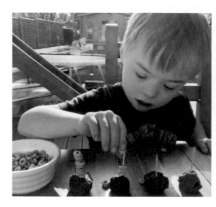

Lockdown home-school 'fun'!
Oscar painstakingly placing Cheerios
on cocktail sticks.
(23 March 2020)

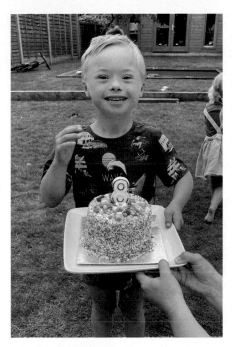

A colourful cake for Oscar's eighth birthday.
(7 July 2020)

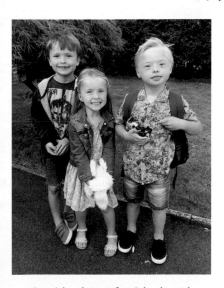

Oscar's last day at Infant School – with
Alfie and Flo.
(21 July 2020)

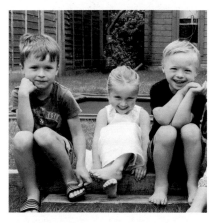

Sitting on the steps – summertime at home.
Oscar with Alfie and Flo.
(28 July 2020)

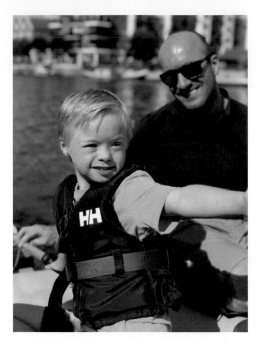

Oscar and Chris boating on the Thames.
(2 August 2020)

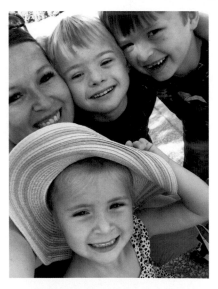

Me, Oscar, Alfie and Flo, on holiday
in Switzerland.
(8 August 2020)

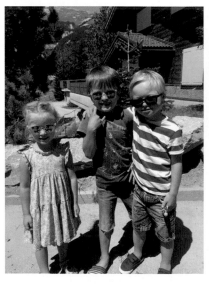

Summer sunshine and sunglasses in
Switzerland: Flo, Alfie and Oscar on holiday.
(9 August 2020)

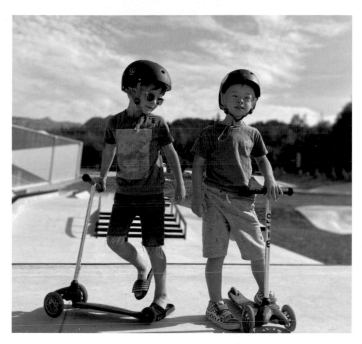

Scooter squad – brothers together, Alfie and Oscar.
(10 August 2020)

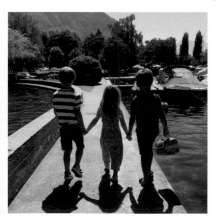

Long summer days on Lake Geneva –
Oscar, Flo and Alfie.
(21 August 2020)

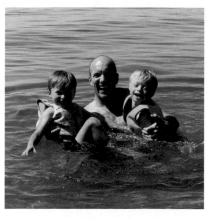

Chris with Alfie and Oscar, swimming in
Lake Geneva.
(21 August 2020)

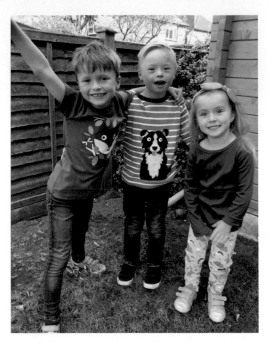

Alfie, Oscar and Flo modelling for sustainable, organic clothes company Frugi.
(27 September 2020)

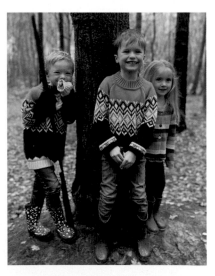

More modelling of Frugi's colourful clothes.
(14 November 2020)

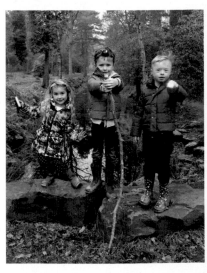

A bright new start in the woods –
New Year's Day, 2021.
(1 January 2021)

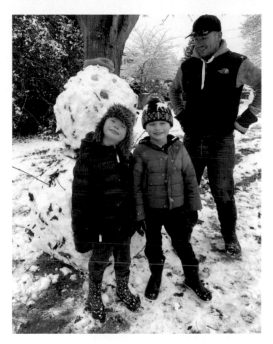

Oscar, Alfie, Chris and snowman.
(24 January 2021)

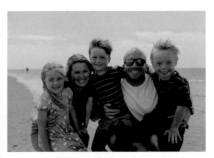

Photograph by www.jessicaisherwoodphotography.co.uk

On the beach at Thornton-Cleveleys,
Lancashire.
(2 June 2021)

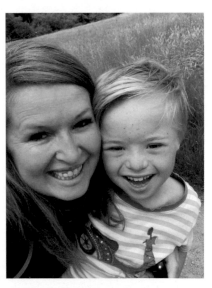

Oscar and me on the common near our home.
(2 July 2021)

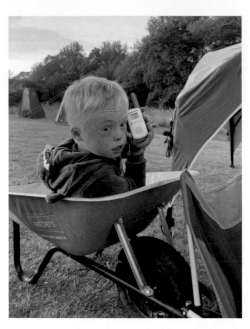

Oscar keeping in touch from his wheelbarrow. A summer evening, camping with friends.
(23 July 2021)

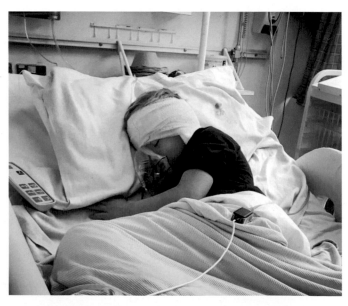

Oscar asleep in hospital following more cholesteatoma surgery.
(29 October 2021)

I don't know why a routine sleep study made me feel like bursting into tears. Oscar had been through far worse in the six years he'd been on this earth, right? He'd been through far, far worse procedures than simply being hooked up to a few wires, probes and beepy machines overnight, for goodness sake. But there was something about a sleep study and the stress and anxiety he goes through to get hooked up to all the above and it had been quite the ordeal this time as he'd got so, so cross with me about it. That always makes me want to cry. And not just for him by the way. For me, too. I mean, obviously I didn't because I'm aware that in the grand scheme of things, there are far, far, FAR worse things that he, or we, might have to go through, but in the interest of being open and honest, occasionally in these situations, I couldn't help thinking, life's a bit shit sometimes.

And no matter how tough you think you are, there are times when being a mum and all the natural instincts that go hand in hand with that title, well, they creep up on you out of nowhere and remind you that being a mummy is tough at times. And it's not just the day-to-day hardcore bits about being a mum because we are all, no matter what our situation, tested by that every day. It's the love stuff, the all-encompassing deep love you feel when your child must go through something you wish they didn't have to. That was what the lump in my throat was earlier. When I'd taken a big, deep breath and not wanted the nurse to see me well up. That was what that was. It wasn't anything else but love. And occasionally, no matter how many times you think you've got this, the love stuff knocks you sideways.

He was asleep now and, although you couldn't see, underneath his PJs he'd been prepped for the study. By this time tomorrow he would have forgiven me for bringing him there, I was sure, but there we were, lying in the darkness. I was trying desperately hard not to make a peep because then he'd know I was there and start getting cross again. There we lay, in silence, wishing the night to be over. Thankfully, the sleep study went well. He woke a couple of times, which was to be expected, but he coped brilliantly, managing to stay asleep for most of the night. It was found that he doesn't have sleep apnoea, so he now has no excuse for waking most nights, but it was good to know that his oxygen levels weren't dipping while he slept. The last time we'd been to get Oscar's heart checked, he had lost it. This is never helpful when an echocardiogram, echo for short, or an ECG (electrocardiogram) is being performed, as the patient needs to remain as still as possible. We had discussed with his consultant that, in order to get a good reading, performing the echo under sedation might be a better shout. So, after his sleep study, we'd walked to the other side of the hospital and Oz had an echo under sedation. This approach seemed a much better idea as he was woozy throughout and kept very calm and still. However, we found out that his lungs were still under strain (pulmonary hypertension), and we'd have to wait another month to hear what his consultants' plan for him would be. The doctor I spoke to that day said there was no urgency, but there were three possible courses of action. The doctors could either:

1. Just keep an eye on it and see how it went over time.
2. Prescribe medication to try to lower the pulmonary hypertension.
3. Perform keyhole surgery through the groin to try to restore blood flow to the lungs.

The good news was that he'd not been showing any signs of distress and that his oxygen levels and blood pressure were within the normal range, but it was still another hurdle we might have to face in the future. So not the best news, but not the worst either. We would see what his consultant had to say and take it from there. I will say, though, that sitting on a hospital ward that morning and talking to other parents certainly puts things into perspective. I met a beautiful little girl and her mother who had had five bouts of open-heart surgery, the last of which had been a complete heart transplant. Listening to the mother's story and all that she and her daughter had been through completely floored me. The little girl sounded like she was doing well now, but if you want real examples of inspiring strength, spend some time on the children's ward of the Brompton Hospital.

* * * *

That summer, we went up to stay with my sister and her two little girls in Norwich. It had been a miserable day, so we headed to Soft-Play Hell. I've always called it that as it was honestly my least favourite thing to do with my kids, yet they loved it and on a grey and murky day, what else was there to do? We'd spent the best part of the first hour waiting in line because the entire population of Norwich had had the same idea as us. In hindsight, I knew that soft play on a rainy day in the summer holidays was a terrible idea and that soft play with an hour wait, where the kids were getting worked up standing in line, was almost definitely not going to end well.

I'd felt proud initially, as for the first half an hour or so once we'd got in Oscar had played beautifully. My niece, who is nine months older than Oscar, had gone around with him, making sure he was okay and even she had commented on how well he was doing. However, as time went by, he appeared to be getting more and more excited and with that excitement it was apparent that everything was becoming a bit more physical. It was nothing major. There would have been a time a few years before when soft play would have been prime time for him to bite someone. This was nothing like that! This time it was just the occasional tap on the head or slap on the back when other kids came past him. There was never any malice in it; he meant no harm. I think it was just his way of getting their attention. But I could see that these kids were starting to get cross with him. Not only were they getting cross, but some had cried and as I looked on – unable to get to him as he was so high up now and trying to get anywhere at speed in soft play, well, you just can't, right? – it felt like these kids were seeking out their parents to tell them about the 'naughty boy'.

I felt like I played it right. I made sure he found each child again and asked him to sign, 'Sorry.' I made a point of trying to figure out who the child's parent was and to apologise to them too. I spoke to Oscar about what he'd done, told him it was unacceptable. I took him off the equipment to give him some time out and told him we would leave if he continued. But I could feel groups of people starting to stare and to make comments around me. And you know what, some days I would have sucked it up. I would have taken a big, deep breath and remembered that even kids without additional needs can act like bell ends too. Even without any diagnosis, they behave inappropriately and aren't very nice. I would have told Oscar to carry on playing, shadowed him, not leaving his side. But some days, when it all gets just a little too much, I get up and leave. I felt their eyes burning into the back of my head, watching me, watching him and I knew that our time there was coming to an end. Just as I felt we'd both had enough, I sensed a mother and her child hovering, ready to speak to me. As I turned, the woman said to her daughter, 'Sweetie, are you okay?' I knew the reason they were there. The mother wanted me to know what Oscar had done. So, as soon as I realised, I asked if Oscar had hurt her, and the girl said that he'd smacked her arm. I explained that Oscar finds it hard to talk, so sometimes that was his way of communicating. I told her that he doesn't always know his own strength and gets excited so sometimes it can come across that he's being horrible. She smiled and said she understood, but then, as I was gathering all my things to leave, I could sense another table of women and their kids all looking over and talking about us. I scooped Oscar up in my arms, bowed my head and left. For the record, I got the stares. I got the whispering to one another and the need to tell me what my little boy had done to their child. But for future reference, as a mum of a child with additional needs, all any of us want for our kids is for them to enjoy the same experiences as the next. We want our child to have fun just like everyone else's. Sometimes it works, sometimes it doesn't. But we've got to try these things for our kids to grow. On days like this one, however, when it all went t*ts up, sometimes we do just leave. Any parent of a child like Oscar is simply trying their best. My anxiety skyrocketed so high in there that I decided it was best to sit in my car and wait for the others. Oscar was sitting behind me, tucking into his lunch, watching an episode of *Paw Patrol* on his iPad, completely and utterly oblivious to the tears streaming down my face.

* * * *

'Mummy?' said Alfie one day, walking in from the garden, where he'd been playing with Oscar and Flo. 'What happened to Oggie's voice? He's lost it. He can't talk to me.'

'What do you mean?' I asked, not expecting the answer he was about to give.

'He doesn't talk to me. Flo does.'

Up until now, I'd always said that both Alfie and Flo had never once questioned anything to do with Oscar. To them, he'd just been Oggie, their big brother. And even when they're beating ten tonnes of cr*p out of each other (they're all as bad as each other with the play-fighting thing) they really do adore one another. But over the summer there'd been a shift in Alfie. He hadn't been asking more questions, but Chris and I had both noticed that he was picking up on a lot more.

Alfie had taken a sudden interest in Oscar's safety and wanted to protect him. If Oscar got too close to a road, Alfie would warn us that he might get squashed by a car. If he'd been eating too many sweets, Alfie would announce that Oscar would get poorly (I mean, they're both things I've said, but he's not meant to be the parent here). Or the time Oscar decided to jump over the barrier fencing on Cromer seafront and lower himself down to the beach (I'm not talking a sheer drop, but I'm not sure many other people would make the jump), and Alfie just about lost his tiny mind that Oggie had fallen. He hadn't; he'd jumped, but Alfie was the first one to find the steps down to the beach and run at speed to 'rescue him'. I appreciate that I'm making myself out to be THE lamest parent here, but, in my defence, I'll say it again, this kid was FAST!!!! Anyway, because of all this, the over-cautious brother thing, mixed with the 'why does Oscar do the things he does' musings, now mixed with the 'Oggie's lost his voice' chat (because Oscar doesn't strike up conversations or often answer with anything other than a yes or a no) plus the fact that Alfie was about to start school that week, we decided we should probably address it because, if another child were to ask Alfie why Oscar is the way he is, he'd then be able to answer.

So, we sat him down. It wasn't too serious. We didn't spend too much time dwelling on it. It went something along the lines of, 'Oscar has Down syndrome, which means it's taking him a bit longer to talk and learn stuff, but he'll get there in his own time.' We also had a book we read to him to help him better understand, 'My friend has Down's syndrome', and although it wasn't a light-bulb moment, we think he came away from our conversation understanding things a little better than he had before.

Blog Comments

'My daughter has had two open-heart surgeries in Bristol children's hospital and her surgeon "Mr Parry" I would consider the greatest man on earth for what he has done for her.'

Kayleigh Challenger Gillbert

'I haven't had a child with DS, but I am a midwife who has looked after many families who have had babies with DS. . . many who weren't expecting it at all, those families that are shocked, crushed, don't know what to do or where to turn. Some who already had the diagnosis and were ready to set out on their path as a family, navigating their

---

beautiful babies' lives and knowing they would just do the best for their baby. All the families I care for are amazing in their own ways and being able to support, encourage and hold the hands of those going through diagnoses, or finding out at delivery is such a rewarding thing for us. Being able to watch those people become a family, helping them in their first few weeks to build that bond and guide them on their journeys with their beautiful bonny babies is just incredible. I am extremely lucky and thankful for my career and the people it allows me to meet.'

Amy Louise

'The paediatrician who delivered the diagnosis to us when Sophie was minutes old was so congratulatory and positive about what her life could be. His language was neutral, he spoke about her like any other baby and really set the tone for the start of our life as a new family of three. I wrote him a letter to say how much his contribution meant to us. We think about him a lot.'

@321_mum

13

Strategies to Smooth the Transition to School

'Note to self – Everything will be okay'
Unknown

Alfie settled into school well. He'd never been a child who'd liked change, but despite missing his key worker from preschool, the first week had gone well. He was on half days for a while as the school's policy was to break the new reception children in gently. And as we were walking back up to school one afternoon to collect Oscar, Alfie and I had a little chat.

Me: 'Did you see Oscar at school earlier, Alfie?'
Alfie: 'Yes, in the playground.'
Me: 'Did you guys play together?'
Alfie: 'I tried.'
Me: 'You tried?'
[Long pause]
Alfie: 'Mummy, I don't have a best friend.'
Me: 'That's okay, you've only just started school, Alfie. You'll make new friends soon.'
[Another long pause]

Alfie: 'Mummy, I don't have a best friend, but Oggar
         has two best friends, a boy and a girl. No one
         played with me.'

And whilst in just that last sentence alone, my heart
broke for my youngest boy, my heart literally exploded
with happiness for my older son. And that, in a nutshell,
sums up the rollercoaster of parenthood, with its highs
and lows.

* * * *

Oscar and I took a trip to London for an appointment
with his heart consultant at the Royal Brompton
Hospital. As Oscar had had the overnight sleep study
done at the hospital, as well as an echo and an ECG, his
consultant wanted to discuss with Chris and me their
plan for Oscar.

They'd been really happy with the pictures they had
been able to take from the echo and the ECG and had been
able to see that although one of the valves had a slight
leak, which may have been a cause of Oscar's pulmonary
hypertension, it wasn't sufficient to warrant medication or
surgery, which had been discussed previously, so we were
really happy with that news.

However, something we weren't expecting to hear, and I
really must remember never to let my guard down with this
kid, was that the sleep study had flagged up that his CO_2
levels were raised, which meant he was showing abnormal
sleep patterns. They decided to refer him to a respiratory
consultant to discuss what she wanted to do about it. So,
not only did we have another consultant to add to the list,
we had more appointments and more trips to London.

This meant that potentially Oscar would need to wear a CPAP (continuous positive airway pressure) mask at night to keep his airways clear. Although it felt like yet another blow, I was wondering if this now explained why Oscar's sleep had been so up and down over the past few years.

They'd also advised that he needed another videofluoroscopy done – the last one had been three years ago – to see what had been going on with his silent aspirating, which could also have been causing the pulmonary hypertension. Before his appointment, we had a bit of spare time, so we went and sat in the gardens next to the hospital. Oscar's open-heart surgery had been five years ago (he was now six) and I will always remember sitting in NICU back then, waiting for him to wake up and looking out of the window, down into the gardens. I vividly remembered thinking that everyone down there seemed as if they didn't have a care in the world. Of course, I know that's not true, for how do any of us know what each of us is dealing with. But, sitting in that garden that day with Oscar, enjoying the sunshine, I wondered if anyone was looking down at us. I'd never been one to sugar-coat things and, although the news that day hadn't been great, if wearing a CPAP mask at night was the worst we'd have to deal with, then we'd take that, I thought.

* * * *

Sometimes people say stupid things. And that's not me meaning to sound like an arsehole, but there have been times over the past nine years when I have been truly perplexed by some of the stuff that comes out of other people's mouths. The other day, having said I had three children, someone asked me if ALL my kids had Down syndrome. I mean, I know it happens occasionally but seriously, three times over??? I'm pretty sure I'd start doing the lottery if that was the case. What'd be the chances?

I also overheard someone say the other day that 'children who have additional needs come from dysfunctional families'. I guess I sort of got what she was getting at (I'm not denying that there will be a percentage who do), but a massive generalisation, don't you think? DS is something that occurs from conception. It's plain and simple science. It's got nothing to do with whether Oscar comes from a crack den or anywhere like that. (He doesn't, obviously.)

A lot of the time, I let this stuff wash over me. What's the point in getting your knickers in a twist about stuff other people say or think? I never believe that it's out of malice; usually I suspect a lack of education or knowledge about the issue.

One of the things that does get my back up, though, is when people talk about siblings and how it's so unfair on them. Sure, from time to time, Alfie and Flo don't always get our full attention, but there are also times when either or both of them take up way more of our time and energy than Oz. When Oscar feels relaxed with someone, he'll take their hand, sit still and play with their fingers. It's something he's done since he was little, and he does it both when he's feeling calm or when he's after a bit of comfort. I walked in to find him and Flo sitting like that the other day and you only have to look at their relationship to know that there is no suffering or burdening of Flo going on. There's nothing unfair about having Oscar as a sibling. Nothing at all.

* * * *

Notoriously, at this time of year, there were a lot of parents of little ones who happen to have Down syndrome wondering how their child was really getting on, having transitioned to school and into reception. Of course, as a parent of a child with additional needs in a mainstream setting, we probably get more feedback than others, via TAs, teachers and communication books. But, unlike other children their age, our kids may not have the verbal communication skills to be able to articulate that they're not happy, not enjoying school or are struggling with the transition. We have to rely solely on a feeling we get from our children because they haven't necessarily got the words to tell us how they're feeling. Remembering when Oscar had started in reception, I cannot fault his school for how they accommodated his transition. If things weren't working, they came up with strategies and solutions to make it work for Oscar, and, by all accounts, they carry on doing so, ensuring that he continues to make progress. Over the last couple of weeks, however, I had had a handful of messages from parents of children who'd just started school, telling me that their children had been excluded from assemblies because they hadn't been able to sit still for the fifteen-minute duration or that they'd been excluded from class because they'd been 'naughty'. Others told me their child had uncharacteristically lashed out at other children in the class and that their child and they had been so upset

It's a big deal for any child starting school – I'd learnt this over the last few weeks with Alfie – but potentially much more so for kids who have additional needs. It's a learning curve for all involved and I believe it's so important to keep communicating with your child's SENCO at the school and to express your concerns if you have any. The only way things can work is if everyone's on the same page and, ultimately, if the school wants to make it work. While I'm not saying Oscar has made huge leaps forward from an academic point of view – that's still very much a work in progress – he had made huge leaps in progress both socially and emotionally.

Oscar had had a little boy come round to our house for a play date. Watching them play with our Paw Patrol figures and vehicles together, jump on the trampoline with one another, and sit having tea together there may have been only a few exchanges of words on Oscar's part, but the friendship they had formed was just so lovely to see. And then at a birthday party of one of his peers, Oscar was very much a part of the group, having just the best time with his friends. It's not often as a mum that I'd get to see that side of things. Like I've said, he couldn't tell me who he'd played with or who'd made his day. But watching him with his friends that weekend reaffirmed for me that, whilst I had no idea how long he would last in a mainstream setting, right then and there he was doing just fine.

The school and I worked together to come up with some ideas about how they could best support Oscar. I have put together some strategies that helped Oscar and others make a smooth transition into education.

Timetabled sensory session
When Oscar was in reception, he would have a session in the hall first thing in the morning. It also included other children in the school who potentially had sensory issues. They'd play sensory games like bouncing on balls, rolling themselves up in mats etc. basically to give them a chance

to expend some energy and channel it properly before sitting down to focus on working in the classroom.

Movement breaks
Oscar's TAs would assess on a day-to-day basis when they felt he was getting fidgety or restless. They would then take him outside, just for a few minutes, which again got rid of some excess energy.

Hot spot
Initially, Oscar struggled to sit still during 'carpet time'. So, they created a 'hot spot' that they could move around, ideally closer to the teacher so he could see/hear.

Heavy backpack
An OT suggested that if he was struggling to focus he should put on a little backpack that was weighted, or to give him a 'job' like carrying a pile of books from one classroom to the next, to bring him back down and ground him. (The weight of both would help with this.)

Leader of the line
A friend's little boy struggled with the transition of going from the playground back into the classroom so they gave him the job of leading the line back inside each time. It gave him something to focus on and a sense of purpose.

Emotion spoons
Another friend's little boy loved playing with wooden spoons and so, for the times he had trouble expressing emotions, she had some 'emotion' spoons made up. On them were various

faces that he could pick out and hold up to show how he was feeling (happy, sad, scared, excited etc.).

Visual timetable
A visual is great for any child, but perhaps more so for children with additional needs. For a child to see in sequence what's going to be happening on a visual cue card really helps ease anxieties.

Now-and-next board
This was something that we introduced back in nursery. It showed what activity was to be carried out first and, once completed, showed what would happen afterwards. A board like this is great for getting kids to do something they're a little more reluctant to do first by showing them the fun thing that would be coming next.

Something to play with in assembly
Occasionally, if the TA picked up that Oscar was having an unsettled morning, she would give him something to play with in assembly to keep him sitting down and focused. It wasn't anything that made a noise that would distract others, just some sort of sensory toy that would fit in the palm of his hand.

Physical contact during carpet time
Initially, when Oscar started school, he couldn't sit on the carpet for long at all. His TA would have to sit behind him with her legs to the side of him, so he couldn't escape. As time went on, she gradually shuffled back so that, in the end, Oscar was able to sit independently for extended

periods of time and could be left, while she busied herself with other tasks. He needed the support to start with, but I guess by then, he had proved he could do it without support in place.

Involving friends in targets
Oscar loved working with other children, so sometimes he would work with classmates on his targets. He loved that he got to 'play' (learn) with his friends, and they loved helping Oscar with his adapted curriculum.

ABC behaviour chart
This is the theory that all behaviour happens as a response to something that has occurred. For example, a child doesn't usually just lash out for no reason. The ABC theory seeks to break down what happened before the incident, what actually happened and what happened as a consequence. It's a great way for professionals to try to understand a child and his or her needs better.

STOP
When a child is too tactile with their peers (even Oscar loves to give a good hug at times), teaching the child who is being touched or hugged to say and sign, 'Stop,' in a clear voice, should hopefully put a stop to any unwanted attention.

We had been having ongoing battles with Surrey County Council (SCC) to ensure the speech and language and occupational therapy provision specified in Oscar's EHCP was carried out. The EHCP was introduced in September

2014, in place of the old 'Statement'. It is a document which sets out the education, health and social care needs of a child or young person and specifies the support that is necessary to cater for those needs.

When Oscar started school, we, along with so many other parents of children with additional needs, fought long and hard to get what we felt he needed in his EHCP. This was to cover the number of hours of 1:1 support we felt he needed in school, along with the speech and language therapy (SALT) and occupational therapy (OT) provision. I'd spent hours filling in forms, collating reports from health-care professionals who had worked with Oscar, going back and forth with the local authority, even going down the route of mediation or a tribunal because at first they wouldn't give us what we knew Oscar needed. The case was thrown out literally a few days before we were supposed to go to court and the local authority did, in the end, give him everything we'd asked for. But it was one of the most stressful times I'd had to date, worrying if Oscar was going to be properly supported in school, or not. However, here we were, two years down the line and what had started so well, with the county council carrying out their side of the agreement, had begun to go wrong. Over the last term or so in reception, I'd noticed that Oscar's OT provision was not being fulfilled.

Having been awarded almost weekly speech and language therapy, meaning that up until this point a SALT had been going in to school to see Oscar each week and delivering 1:1 therapy sessions (with Oscar's TA present), I was interested to see how this was going to pan out. When he'd started school, having been allocated his EHCP, the council said they didn't have the resources to cover the amount of SALT awarded so outsourced a private speech therapist, at additional cost to themselves, to deliver his sessions. That part of it worked brilliantly, but in July that year, his private SALT told me that the council had terminated her contract with Oscar and, from the beginning of the following academic year, he would be given an NHS SALT, employed directly by them. You can imagine my reservations.

When we were half-way through week five of his first term in Year 1, he hadn't yet seen an OT and his SALT had delivered only one direct therapy session. In defence of his new OT, we had spoken on the phone and she was apparently wanting to go in to see Oscar 'soon'. At the end of the previous term, I had contacted our case officer to bring to their attention that the OT provision had not been carried out as required and to remind them that an EHCP is a legally binding document (that I had fought b****y hard for), and that I would not be taking this lightly. I said that if the provision wasn't rectified in future, I would be contacting my local government ombudsman to take things further, which, funnily enough, got everyone moving again. But my point here is why did everything have to be a constant fight? What would happen to those children whose parents hadn't got the fight in them, either because they didn't understand the system or weren't sufficiently confident or articulate to drive things forward. If Oscar had been in a specialist school surely he would be costing the local authority a lot more money than he was now? Therefore, surely, they'd want to make it work. I closely monitored when his SALT and OT went in to school to see Oscar that term. And while I wasn't disputing the fact that it must be hard for them to manage all the children eligible for assistance when they are short of funding, resources and therapists, that wasn't really the point. I'd heard that

Surrey County Council had cut £21 million from the budget for children with SEN, which was maddening. Had they felt that the education of those children who needed support was worth less than the next child? I desperately hoped not.

Blog Comments

'When an inquisitive supermarket check-out lady asked about Bailey's NG tube, I explained that Bailey had DS and a cardiac issue, which meant she needed help with feeding, she replied, "Oh! She's still beautiful though!"'

Nic Edginton

'"If you have this baby it will end up in an institution" (paediatric consultant, 2014).
"If there's a birth emergency, do you want it resuscitated" (neonatal paediatrician, 2014).'

Cath Erine

'I was asked by a random stranger while on a train journey, did I not think of having a termination. She then went on to say she was a teacher.'

Samantha Moss

14

Couch to 5k

'*If you never try, you'll never know*'
Unknown

During the summer, I'd found myself feeling flat. I'd realised it was nothing to do with Oscar or the others, it was just me. I think the kids were getting older and somewhere along the way, I'd lost myself a little, and my sense of purpose. Aside from the odd dance class, I hadn't been doing anything in the way of exercise and that was having a big impact on my mental health. The trouble is, with the interrupted nights and early mornings, it felt like a vicious circle. I was reaching for the biscuits mid-morning because I was so shattered, putting on weight and then feeling too lethargic to exercise.

But something shifted in September, and I started Couch to 5K. I'm not going to lie, I absolutely hated it when I was doing it, but I realised quite quickly that afterwards I felt great. It didn't take that long and yet the sense of achievement I had after running lasted for quite some time. So, in October, I decided to do something I could never have imagined doing previously. I signed up for the London Marathon to raise money for the Down's Syndrome Association. It might sound like a crazy thing to have done, especially for a chubby mum of three, who was a non-runner, but I knew that setting myself a goal and telling people, for example, my followers on my social media platforms, would make me accountable. I knew that if I talked about it online, people would get behind me and sponsor me (after all, so many who take the time to follow me have some sort of link to DS, but if not, many have simply fallen in love with Oscar). I also knew that telling people I was running the marathon would mean that I had to do it. I am many things, but a quitter is not one of them!

That October I posted that I was running for the Down's Syndrome Association. I spoke about the fact that when I was running, I was mostly muttering FML (F**k my life!) under my breath (that's when I managed to catch my breath), but that running gave me a sense of purpose again. I spoke of all the reasons I wanted to do it. I mentioned that my friend Steph had done it the year before and she'd said it'd be a cool thing to say I'd done it in my fortieth year. And honestly, it gave me something to focus on when the boys were at school, and Flo was at preschool. It was also around that time that I was writing my first book, so I was busy. But looking back, although hard, it was honestly one of the most exhilarating and liberating things I have ever done. I trained hard. I'm not talking hardcore runner-style hard, but I'd go out three times a week, gradually increasing my distance and slowly building up my stamina. More on that later.

* * * *

I'd come across a post on Instagram written by a midwife, who was asking whether it was right that we share our experiences of pregnancy and birth if they have been particularly traumatic. She was pondering whether it was fair on unassuming pregnant women to be reading them as it might fuel their anxieties? I gave my opinion and wrote a bit about what I did on my page. I wrote about *my* outcome with Oscar and let the midwife and other readers know that, while I totally appreciated that everyone has the right to choose whether to screen for DS, I felt that if a woman gets an unexpected diagnosis, either prenatally or post-natally, to my mind it's so important that health-care professionals remain unbiased and mindful of not trying to project their own opinions as to what life might be like with a child who happens to have DS, and that they absolutely shouldn't ever push a woman into having a termination. I mean, this sounds like I went off on a tangent, but it was relevant within the thread.

A few minutes after I'd left my comment, a student midwife replied to me saying that while she understood what I was saying to a degree, she also wanted to let me know that if *she* was delivering a diagnosis of DS, she too would apologise. She then launched into a spiel about how important it is for women to have the choice, even if it is late in their pregnancy. For the record, I'm pro-choice and totally agree that everyone should be free to make their own choice.

As I was reading her comment, I felt so sad that this was a student midwife. Students are usually the ones who are open to change, the ones who seem shocked to hear about the abortion rates related to DS and so on. Students are usually the ones who soak everything up, digest it and then tell us they understand. I felt gutted that she'd seemed so set on testing for DS because it was apparent to me that she viewed DS as a bad thing. I know we're not going to be able to change everyone's mind, but reading her comments revealed the stark reality that there is still so much unconscious bias, even amongst health-care professionals.

A few days later, I received the following message. And although I loved that this woman was strong enough to know her own mind, I just felt so very sad – again – that this midwife had kept on, knowing that she was standing strong in what she believed in.

Hi Sarah,

You were the first person I wanted to share this with. I hope you don't mind!

My daughter is expecting her first baby, a little girl due in January. She was telling me today that at one of her antenatal appointments earlier in the pregnancy, she had been offered screening for Down's Syndrome. My daughter declined the screening with the thoughts that, she is having a baby – full stop. What came after is quite honestly shocking. She was then questioned as to whether she understood what it means to have a baby with Down's Syndrome and what they could 'do' if the screening revealed she had DS. Now I don't know if my daughter was treated this way as she is a young mum, and if it would have been different for an older parent?!? I am just so proud of my girl who stood up for herself and her baby. After seeing you making a difference to language being used by professionals, I probably naively thought it would be wider spread. Keep up your fantastic work.

xx

In this country, around ninety per cent of women who find out they're expecting a baby with DS choose to terminate. I have been contacted so many times by women saying that, having found out the baby they're carrying does indeed have DS, and even though they've categorically stated they DO NOT wish to terminate, they are repeatedly asked whether they have changed their minds and are sometimes pushed into terminating. Again, in this country, if it's found that you're carrying a baby who happens to have DS, by law you can terminate your pregnancy up until thirty-nine weeks and six days, that is one day short of full term. So that's why I keep sharing our story and I'll keep commenting on other people's posts, because I really do hope that one day, things will change.

* * * *

Oscar and I had spent the afternoon at the Royal Brompton Hospital, in London. After having a sleep study done a few months ago, which had found that Oscar's CO_2 levels were dipping more than they'd like, they'd said he had abnormal sleep patterns and they wanted to investigate why. He'd been referred to a respiratory consultant, who asked me to describe a typical night's sleep for Oscar to try to establish what might be causing his abnormal sleep patterns. At this time, Oscar could wake once or twice a night, but on a bad night, he could be up around six times. He would also always wake early every day, between 4.30

and 5 a.m. which had taken its toll over the years. We always just assumed that this was normal for Oscar, but his consultant thought that it could be reflux, which is always worse when one lies down. Oscar had a chest X-ray done while we were there and, although one lung looked clear, the other had definite shadowing, and appeared to be under strain.

As a result of this, we decided to try him on some reflux medication for a one-month period to see if his sleep improved. Then, after that month, we'd take him off it to see if he went back to his normal (dreadful) sleep pattern. We were going to be heading back up to the Royal Brompton Hospital at the beginning of the following month to the Speech and Language department, who would be looking at his silent aspirating, and they would do a test for reflux at the same time.

It sometimes felt never-ending. Don't get me wrong, it wasn't the worst thing that could have happened, but it always felt as if there was something else being added to the appointment list, which could at times be disheartening. At this stage, though, had the new reflux medication worked, I would obviously have stopped my moaning about extra hospital appointments and been thrilled. Actual SLEEP!!!!!! I'm not sure I could even remember what that was!!!!

* * * *

Back when I'd first had Oscar, after the initial feelings of 'this wasn't the way I had imagined our lives going', I remember that afterwards I'd felt like I wanted to be around other people who were experiencing what I was feeling. I guess I wanted to actually seek out those others who had felt all that stuff, but come out the other side. I'm not denying there is a huge network of support through the online community – forums, blogs and social media pages – but for us, getting involved in a local DS support group was a lifeline at the time.

I already had a connection to my local one, PSDS (Providing Support for Children with DS and their families), in that I was teaching a dance/drama class for them once a week, so I guess, for me, it was easier to reach out to them. Many of the DS support groups across the country run early development sessions. This is often subsidised by a charity and the focus is usually on speech and language. There has been a huge amount of research done to prove that early intervention with our kids helps greatly. Like any child, the more we put into them, the more likely they are to achieve. The groups also offer social opportunities for the whole family, which I think has been important for both Alfie and Flo, to grow up knowing other kids in the same situation. If you had told me when I'd had Oz that some of my closest friends would be other parents of kids who happen to have DS, I would have scoffed, I know I would. But I cannot tell you how invaluable peer support for parents in these groups is.

I love the fact that Oscar is in a mainstream setting and has friendships within the class. But I think it's been lovely for Oscar to have other friends outside of school, who, like him, also happen to have DS. Many of the groups run youth clubs, sports clubs and so on, and I guess some might feel that as kids get older and it's potentially not so easy for them to attend mainstream groups, this becomes more important for them. Many groups offer training to parents, nurseries and schools, which they'd be unlikely to be able to access anywhere else, especially such specialist expertise.

I don't think I need to mention the lack of funding and resources for local councils again, but these groups need *active* members for them to continue to run. That means members who contribute, not just money, but time and energy. Groups simply can't survive without members, but to be flourishing, dynamic groups, they need people to support them and to help run them.

I'd spoken at a DS support group networking event hosted by Nicola Enoch, who runs the website PADS (Positive About Down Syndrome) and, as I'd sat and listened to others talk, what stood out for me was what a passionate group of men and women they are. Not only was it obvious that they all had so much knowledge, experience and a desire to help, but none of them were sitting around moaning about life. It was apparent to me that it was about ensuring our kids are given every opportunity. So, if you're reading this, new to this particular journey and thinking about reaching out locally to see what's available if you're looking for a bit of extra support, I can promise you, we have never looked back from having joined a group.

* * * *

Around this time, it felt like we were up and down to London a lot. Oscar had the day off school as he had a couple of appointments at the Royal Brompton Hospital again. His first appointment was to assess his swallowing, as they had previously suspected that he had reflux, but the medication for this had not worked; and the second was to meet with a speech therapist who specialised in eating and drinking. His lungs had been under strain and he was showing signs of mild pulmonary hypertension. At that point, it wasn't a massive deal, but, if left, it could have a big impact on how long he's on this earth for. He had his videofluoroscopy done. This is a procedure where they give him a special liquid to drink and then take an X-ray video to see where the drink is going when he swallows. They could see almost immediately that it was going into his windpipe which we thought might be happening, which was why he'd always had a thickener in his drink. We then tried it with a drink that I'd made up for him, with the thickener in it, and once again, to our surprise this time, we saw some seep into his windpipe.

Oscar had been on the thickener since he was three, but a couple of years after being on it, we changed the consistency, so it became less like custard and had more of a syrup-like consistency. To cut a long story short, he should probably never have stopped with the custard-like consistency as he was only assessed by an independent SALT watching him and he appeared to be managing well on the syrup. In hindsight, he should probably have had a videofluoroscopy to check what was actually happening back then. We now had a possible explanation as to why his lungs were under strain and we were given strict instructions to go back to giving him the gloopiest, thickest drinks to try to rectify this. We were also told at the appointment that it could take a year to eighteen months for the lungs to fully recover. You would have had no idea, being around him, that he had this, as I genuinely don't think it affected him day to day, but we were just so grateful that it had been discovered before it did any more damage, and that he'd now be monitored. There are times, as a parent of a child with additional needs, that you can feel like there's been a run of health-related appointments, which can feel frustrating and relentless. But I was just so grateful that Oscar was continuing to get the care he did from our wonderful NHS (the UK's National Health Service), who leave no stone unturned in caring for him.

Blog Comments

'We had the most amazing screening midwife when we had the antenatal diagnosis. She made no presumptions about what we would do and didn't force any views or outdated opinions on us. Just listened to us and spent so much time with us. For me after a couple of weeks knowing the diagnosis, I realised it wasn't the diagnosis but the alternative that some consultants were telling us we had to decide on. Angie, thanks for your kindness and just being there when we needed.'

Despina Papadimitriou

'After Hollie was born, we had the most wonderful health visitor, Carol. She had such a positive impact on how I got my head around it all, with a postnatal diagnosis. It saddens me to say that she passed away only a few years later. I will always remember her and am so grateful for her.'

Laura Egan

'I often think of the nurse in theatre who was with me the whole time while having my planned C-section. We knew our little guy had DS and a significant heart defect. I was doing okay that morning in the lead-up to the section, but as soon as they started to open me up, it was like all the fear of him being on the outside and not protected anymore just

---

came out as they made the incision. I just silently cried the whole way through the surgery, and she wiped the tears from my cheeks with a tissue. She was so caring. After he was born and those anxious few mins while he was checked had passed, he was brought over and placed by my cheek for a couple of minutes while I was being stitched up. She made sure to get those first few pics before he was whisked away by ambulance to the paediatric hospital to get his heart checked. I still think of her often and tried to find her name in my file before I left the hospital but had no luck.'

Rebecca Loughnayne

15

Mainstream or SEN?

Oscar was in Year 1, but at the end of Year 2, if he was to do what most of the children at his school do, he would join the local mainstream junior school, just down the road. At a meeting towards the end of the autumn term, a professional who had worked with Oscar that term (not an employee of the school) looked me straight in the eye and told me that although she knew it wasn't her place to tell me what to do, if I wanted her honest opinion, she believed Oscar would be best suited to a specialist SEN (Special Educational Needs) school from Year 3. As you can imagine, being faced with this out of the blue I'd been quite taken aback. We'd been having a frank and honest discussion about Oscar's development so it was in context and, for the record, I certainly didn't feel any animosity towards the professional in question. She was right: Oscar did struggle with his speech, he was very behind academically, even by the standards of his peers who also happen to have DS and, although he had some lovely little friends in his class, we had been wondering if he'd manage to keep those friendships, or if the children would soon tire of his inability to converse, even on a basic level? Our gut feeling was that Oscar would be better suited to a specialist setting from Year 3, but listening to the professional's thoughts and hearing her confirm what, if we were honest with ourselves, we'd known for a while was very painful. Hearing it said out loud really hurt. And I'm not even sure why it felt like such a blow. I'd certainly understood the benefits to Oscar of attending a SEN school and I knew in my heart that sending your child to a specialist setting isn't some sort of failure. But I felt there was a stigma. I remember very clearly when Oscar was born, having had all these hopes and aspirations for his future, feeling that they were being taken away somehow. The blunt words from the professional felt like a bitter pill to swallow.

When I spoke to a friend about how this had made me feel, she hit the nail on the head when she said we'd been those parents who'd wanted our child to prove everyone wrong, to prove that he could do anything he set his mind to: go to mainstream school; find a job; learn to drive; live alone; find a partner to love, and so on. We'd wanted all those things for him, yet, for some reason, with this potential change of path now, that all felt like it was slipping away. We weren't sure what the future held any more and, whilst I suppose none of us ever really do, regardless of where our children go to school, his felt like a really significant change. Looking back now, I realise that when you're faced with something like this, for me, it felt very much like when we'd found out about Oscar's diagnosis. We were now mourning the loss of that 'normal' again, and that was hard. I think mostly it affected me so badly because I hadn't expected to have to confront this quite so soon. We knew other children with DS much older than Oscar who were thriving in mainstream schools and that's what we'd hoped for for him. But I think maybe we also had a gut feeling at this point that Oscar wasn't thriving; he was just surviving and coasting along. I'll be truthful, this hadn't been what I'd wanted nor how I thought it would go. I knew the only thing that mattered here wasn't how I was feeling, but what was in Oscar's best interests. Ultimately, however I felt about it, Oscar's happiness would be the only successful outcome.

Literally the day after that meeting, when I was still feeling a little bruised from the bashing my heart had taken, I'd gone along to watch Oscar in his school nativity play. Up until this point we'd had mixed success. The first year, Oscar had nailed it. The previous year, not so much. However, this year, with the biggest, broadest grin plastered on his face, he marched up onto that stage, indoors this time, and when it was his turn, he danced his little heart out (bowing repeatedly to the audience's applause). Oh, and Alfie, the boy who up until this point had always outright refused to join in with any sort of performance-based activity, stood centre stage and sang and danced like a little superstar too. Obviously, I had a mini-weep, the type you have when you're half laughing and half bursting with heart-smoshing pride. Oz and his little bro Alf had smashed it out of the park, reminding me once again that life is one mighty big rollercoaster of twists and turns and that these moments are a gentle reminder to us all that whatever happens, it's going to be okay.

* * * *

I'd been invited to St George's Hospital, in Tooting, London, to film a clip for a new online video the senior midwife co-ordinator was putting together about NIPT (non-invasive prenatal testing, a method for determining the likelihood that your baby will be born with certain genetic differences). The training video was to be available to health-care professionals and students who wanted to access further information on NIPT. My role was to give my opinion on the test, but also to give them a little insight into our family.

This is such a subjective matter and opinions on it differ greatly. Some people won't consider the test because, to them, the outcome would be irrelevant; they would keep their baby regardless. Others might want the information, to know ahead of time if their baby has DS in order to prepare, but wouldn't terminate the pregnancy. And others want that information because under no circumstances would they consider having a baby with a disability like Down syndrome.

Knowledge is power and if people feel they want to know, the procedure is something for them to consider. But my beef is that it's not 100 per cent accurate and when it's offered I don't think that's always made clear. NIPT is 98 to 99 per cent effective, which means that for one in a hundred people, the results they receive won't necessarily be correct. Does this mean that some babies being flagged as having a high chance of having DS are being aborted simply on that basis? But my biggest issue with this is the way in which the test is being explained by some, though certainly not all, health-care professionals, the language that is used. The assumption appears to be that just because someone has chosen to have the test they would abort if it were found that their baby was at higher risk of a genetic abnormality. It's not just words like 'risk' being bandied about, but also the fact that in some cases as soon as a woman finds out that she's supposedly expecting a baby who may have DS, they are then handed leaflets about terminations on the spot, without any real attempt to gauge how that woman and her partner might be feeling.

So I said all that to the screening midwife. I said everything I'd wanted to say. But I also told them about Oscar – his life, his family, how much he loves us and how much we love him. I spoke about how one of the best things about having Oscar is watching the dynamic between him, Alfie and Flo, how they love each other completely; also how my opinion on Down syndrome and what it means to have a child who happens to have the condition is so very different now from how I felt during the moments that followed Oscar's diagnosis. I told them how I was wrong in the beginning. I knew I wasn't going to change the minds of a lot of health-care professionals because, the way I see it, is that they only get to see the bad bits. Perhaps by talking about what life is really like with Oscar, I may give others a better understanding. I really hope so.

* * * *

On this morning in January 2019, Oscar had two hours of investigative surgery on his ear, which found that the ear was clear and finally free of the cholesteatoma. He would always have to be monitored and there was obviously a chance that it could grow back, but for now it meant no more surgery and he would just have to be checked as an out-patient at the ENT clinic. There are times when it feels like every time this kid gets a bit of a break, there is yet another setback, so it felt so amazing to get some good news this time. He had had a lot of pain relief during the course of the day and would almost certainly be dosed up on the magic pink stuff that night, but he was home, and we were all happy.

A few weeks after his surgery, Oscar's sleep became particularly disturbed. I went to bed at about 10 p.m. and by 11 p.m. he was awake. Then every hour after that up until 5 a.m. he'd woken up. Some might say I'd been fortunate in that usually he woke up I'd go in to him, give him a bit of reassurance that I was there and he'd drift straight back off to sleep. I didn't usually have to stay with him or lie with him for hours, which I know some people have to do, so for the most part, because I was so exhausted at that time of night, once I was back in our bed, I would fall straight back to sleep.

But this particular night, because he was so full of cold, he just wouldn't go back to sleep. I knew lots of people who let their kids get into bed with them and I am all for that if you all then get a great night's sleep, but on the odd occasion we'd tried it, Oscar would think it was party time and we'd spend the entire night having to tell him it was night-time. So, this night, unable to leave his room because every time I did he'd cry out, I sat in the dark on his bedroom floor. And knowing he just needed to know I was there, I allowed my phone to provide a little bit of light for him to see that.

As I sat there, browsing a page on Facebook for parents of kids who happen to have DS, the first thing I read about was a child who hadn't slept in years, how his parents had been at their wits' end because he hadn't slept for longer than ninety minutes at any one time EVER, and how the respite care that they'd had once a week for the past few years wasn't working out. It was one of those moments, as I sat there in the dark, when I suddenly felt very low. People often say to me that I'm so positive and that I always see the best in every situation, but right then, I couldn't help thinking that there didn't ever seem to be an end to this.

It's not often that I let things get to me like that, but at that time of night, willing Oscar to go back to sleep, I felt cross that this was the card I'd been dealt. I knew there were hundreds of women and men sat with their babies and toddlers across the world, willing them to go back to sleep, soothing them, reassuring them, but I felt bitter that their sleep deprivation was probably going to be short-lived. And in that moment, it all just felt very bleak. Was I still going to be sat on Oscar's bedroom floor in twenty years' time? Of course, in the light of day I would have been fine. I knew that by the following week, once Oscar's cold had gone, things would settle down. I knew that after an early night and Chris getting up with him next time, I'd be okay because that's what we do as parents of kids with additional needs. We acknowledge it's hard, brush ourselves off and we get on with it. People would often ask me how I coped with the broken sleep. I think I coped with it because I consciously chose to be happy. I don't usually allow myself to dwell on my lack of sleep because if I had, I'm not sure I would ever have got out the hole. Some days it was tough. But that didn't mean I loved my child any less. I know it is important for me to acknowledge at times that parenting a child like Oscar is hard, and I make no apology for admitting that.

* * * *

In the eyes of a parent of a child who happens to have DS, a milestone, however small, is always celebrated. I'd taken Oscar to a birthday party one afternoon. It was the first one he'd ever been to on his own. I was there, but when the birthday girl's mum said he'd be fine and to go downstairs and join the rest of the parents, who were all having coffee, completely out of sight of the children, I'd joined them. And as I sat, trying to concentrate on what the other parents were all talking about, my mind was racing: *Would he join in? Would he cause trouble? Was he okay without someone specifically watching him?* It's funny, really, because I imagine it's probably not something parents of typical kids have ever had to think about. By the time they've reached the age of six, I guess they don't give dropping children off at a party for a couple of hours a second thought because of course their children will be okay. But Oscar literally had to have someone with him the entire time. Whether it was Chris or me or a TA at school, there was always someone with him, so leaving him upstairs at the party had been a big old deal. And do you know what? He bloody well did it. He'd joined in. He'd not caused trouble. And even though he'd crept downstairs at one point to check I was still there, once he'd seen me again, he'd gone right back in to the thick of the party-game action. Sometimes for us, progress could feel so unbelievably slow. Some days, I wondered if we'd ever get there. But as I thought about that party, how he'd interacted with his friends, played with them, sat at the table for tea with them (and how he couldn't have cared less whether I was there or not at that point . . . he had cake!!!!) I realised how far we'd come. He was really growing up. It had been so easy to get hung up on milestones and when he was going to make the next leap in progress, but that afternoon reminded me that occasionally our little guy would surprise us with how brilliant he could be.

Hi Sarah,

Yesterday I directed two student doctors to your page, I do hope they follow. You see after eleven days in hospital with my daughter (two of those in ICU) we were finally being discharged and about to leave when a doctor came to our room who I hadn't seen before.

He said he knew I was about to go but would I mind sparing some time so he could bring in some students. I knew we were in a teaching hospital so it's quite common and thinking he wanted to discuss my daughter's reason for being there, I said no problem. It transpired that what he really wanted was to treat her like some kind of circus act, pointing out all the shortcomings of Down Syndrome! He continuously used 'they' like children with DS are all the same. He was suggesting to the students that they should establish facts, and many can be gained by looking around the bedside. He went on to speak about the toys she had around her (I may add all provided and belonging to the hospital) and how they can tell us a lot. He said, 'For a child to be sitting unaided like this, I wouldn't expect to see baby toys so it would suggest developmental delays of some sort'!! They were mostly musical instruments and age-appropriate. Whilst I did stop him in his tracks several times and correct a few things, I found myself really taken aback. He didn't seem keen when I suggested the students look you up and spoke about the great work you do and how they could learn a lot about parent-friendly language! Many things he said were inappropriate and actually incorrect, like telling them that most babies sit unaided by five months and walk at ten months! This is not my first baby, so I am aware of what her delays are, but I certainly don't need them to be pointed out in this way and especially after eleven worrying days and virtually no sleep. I drove home in tears; I still have a migraine! The tears were of frustration as I feel I let her down and let down the DS community as I didn't say enough. I will always be my daughter's number-one ambassador and her generation are driving a sea-change in attitudes, but how sad it is that that change does not have all the medical profession at the forefront of it? Please continue to do what you do; I will endeavour to be more vocal in the future and I'm praying those students look you up.

I received the above message, which I think is so important to highlight. I share it not because I want to call this hospital out, but just to say that ALL of us, every single one of us, should be open to learning from others. This woman felt she hadn't done enough (I can't tell you the number of times I walk away from a situation and think what I COULD have said), but I wanted to reassure her and others that simply trying and showing how passionately you feel about something is all any of us can do.

Blog Comments

'Ben was at mainstream school both for primary and secondary, which was the right choice for him at that time. He thrived at primary school and in the first three years of secondary, then we noticed that his friendships were not the same any more. Yes, everyone was nice to him, but they weren't real friendships. The need for more independence, life skills and friendships were not being met at his mainstream school any more, so post sixteen we chose a SEN school and boy is he thriving.

He's so much happier, so much more independent and has proper friends!!'

Anna Bird

'George repeated reception in mainstream, and it became obvious during that second year that he would not be able to continue into Year 1. It was totally heart-breaking, and I cried because he was going to leave his peers and the mainstream system which we had been told was the way forward. I cried until I realised this move to SEN school was best for him, and my sadness wasn't part of the equation. And it indeed was best. He is happy and thriving. Mainstream would have enhanced his differences and difficulties. We did the right thing, but the initial realisation can be hard.'

Tatty Bowman

'My son is currently in a SEN setting and I know, if he were in mainstream school, they'd not have the time or manpower to be able to help him the way his current school are geared up to do. Sadly ALL areas of the education system are fit to burst, and, I know it's a pipe dream, but if the powers that be completely overhauled the system, reassessed how schools work, updated and redressed the balance so that ALL children (with or without additional needs) would be able to go to a setting that has the ability to help them reach their potential the way they each need it, imagine how that would be?!'

Anon

16

What I'd Tell My Former Self

'When I let go of what I am, I become what I might be'
Lao Tzu

In February 2019, we took the kids skiing. Chris had always been a big skier and we'd gone a few times before we'd had children, but I wasn't a natural. In fact, I think I'd spent most of the time absolutely petrified that I was so completely out of control and likely to go arse over tit at any time that I hadn't found it that enjoyable (the Glühwein après-ski was more my bag). So, we'd decided that starting them young was a must. Oscar was six, Alfie five and Flo just three. Flo hadn't been that keen initially. Going down the training slopes hadn't been the issue, more that she had to negotiate her way up onto the belt to get herself back up to the top and that she'd found hard. We'd signed all three of them up to ski school and every time we left her she'd have a face like thunder or she'd cry because she didn't want to do it. Alfie took to it all like a duck to water and was soon promoted to the more advanced group. And then there was Oz. The kid, who on paper, due to having low muscle tone and developmental delays as a result of his

DS, would probably find this the most difficult. Except, in true Oscar style, he faced the challenge with his usual guts and determination, as he has done with every hurdle, and within minutes, he was gliding down the slopes too.

Chris had decided to stay with Oscar for the lesson. We knew that Oscar had trouble staying on task sometimes and at this stage he also wasn't toilet trained yet (the ongoing toileting journey was still in full swing). So we'd decided that shadowing him this time would be for the best. I'd looked on, making sure I was out of sight, and noted that when it came to the technique bits, he'd lose interest a little. But when it came to the execution and giving it a go, he did so with energy and enthusiasm, just throwing himself into it. And although his technique may not have been the best, his balance was incredible. Watching him that week, skiing down the training slopes with his little brother and sister, watching them having fun together in the snow, is a memory that will stay with me forever, particularly as it really hadn't ever been something I'd even dared dream about when I'd first had Oscar. The truth is it's not just society which puts limits on what we expect from a child who has DS. Here I'd been, as his mother, fretting over whether skiing would be too much of a challenge for him. And here he was again, proving me wrong and showing me that anything's possible.

When we got back from that ski trip, we found out from a hearing test that Oscar's hearing had deteriorated significantly. It was frustrating because towards the end of the summer his hearing had been great, and they'd reported that it was within normal range. But during the winter, a build-up of congestion from colds and a few ear infections had resulted in moderate hearing loss in both ears. We were also told that he'd need another grommet fitted in one of his ears, so we were awaiting a surgery date for that. In the grand scheme of things, grommets are a walk in the park compared with the massive surgeries he's had, but it was still yet another operation for this little man. With Oscar having had ongoing ear problems from a very early age, I had often wondered if they were the main cause of his speech difficulties. In the summer, when his hearing was great, there still hadn't been much, if any, improvement. We knew that, despite his weekly SALT interventions and all the extra work they were doing with him at school, progress appeared to be slow. People would often ask me how Oscar communicated. At this stage, he had a handful of key words he could say which seemed to enable him to get by, also a selection of Makaton signs. He'd been trying so hard to talk, babbling away at length, with the occasional word in there that I could recognise, but it was all still painfully slow. A mum of an older child who also has DS asked me if I'd 'resigned myself to the fact that this is it now?', in other words that Oscar would probably never talk any more than he did at that stage. It had taken me off guard a little as the question was quite direct and the issue was something that had niggled away at the back of my mind, and continues to do so, but I still had hope. Maybe that was naive, but this couldn't be it, could it? One thing I'd learned over the six years of having Oscar was that all kids who happen to have DS are SO very different. One child might excel in one area in which another is weaker, and vice versa.

We had been told that soon we'd need to start filling in paperwork, eighteen months in advance of when he'd be transitioning, to apply for Oscar's next school. I had spent hours, both online and talking to others in a similar position to us, exploring our options as to which mainstream and

SEN options were available to Oscar. If the truth be told, both Chris and I, despite our instinct that a SEN school would be better, were at a loss. We could see the pros and cons of both, and we agreed you almost wished you could have a crystal ball to see the outcomes of both options. Some weeks I was so certain that mainstream was where Oscar should be, for the friendships he'd formed, because he continued to learn so much from his mainstream peers and because of how hard his school worked to include him in as much of the curriculum as they could, adapting it as necessary so he could be part of the class. I was conscious too that I was being influenced by others who had travelled along our path previously and whose sons and daughters were doing brilliantly in the mainstream system. Listening to them expressing how much of a success mainstream had been for their child and how putting Oscar in a SEN setting might have a detrimental effect on him, felt completely compelling at times. The noise around mainstream versus SEN in our community is a real thing and there is an obvious divide in that some feel that we're failing our kids by sending them down the SEN route and others feel that SEN is for the best. It's such a tough call because what's right for one child with DS is only right for that one child with DS. There isn't a one-size-fits-all approach because all our kids are so very different. I also think that if mainstream works for a child who happens to have DS or not is so dependent on the school and the supporting staff. Do they really want it to work? Are they constantly adapting and differentiating where they need to for that child? Are they wanting to learn more strategies and what works for our kids? Are they going on courses, absorbing information from professionals who have first-hand experience of working with children with DS? Because if the answer to any of those questions is no, I really do think you're fighting a losing battle.

One minute I was convinced that mainstream was where Oscar should be, but then, when he appeared not to be as engaged as he'd been the previous week, or when he was unsettled or a bit less willing to join in, I'd then wonder if continuing down the mainstream route was the right thing for him after all.

Academically, progress had been slow. It felt like he was still working on much the same things as he had been yonks ago, simply because he'd yet to master that something. But then I'd remember what so many people had said, that we shouldn't expect him to be keeping up with his peers anyway, and it's not about the academic side of things, it's about whether he's happy and making any progress, no matter how minuscule the steps might seem. When I'd spoken about SEN settings on my social media pages, the support in favour of them had been overwhelming from those whose children had made the transition themselves. Yet then I would get inundated with private messages, telling me not to sell him short and that mainstream is absolutely where our children should be, because they're capable of so much if channelled correctly and the support is there. I know I shouldn't have been listening to or even asking others what they thought because ultimately it would be Chris's and my decision, but the fact that WE had to make this decision for him and there was a chance that we would get it very wrong, well, that felt like a lot on our shoulders.

One day after school, as we walked past our local children's playground, Oscar, Alfie and Flo asked to go in. I was usually mean. When they asked, I'd say that we couldn't go in because at that time of day it was so busy and trying to keep track of all of them would give me heart palpitations, then we'd leave with me cursing myself for being a d**k for even thinking going into the playground had been a good idea. But this time, in a moment of weakness, I'd agreed. Alfie and Flo were happily playing on the equipment, chatting to friends, but Oscar ran straight to the patch of grass where the older kids were playing football. My first thought, knowing how seriously boys take football, was that the arrival of Oscar wasn't going to go down that well. Some of the bigger boys were from the junior school and so my instinct was to start thinking of ways to get him back into the playground. But as I watched, I realised it wasn't an issue at all. Some of the boys had shouted hello when he'd come over and others were happily passing him the ball. None of them got cross when he went in for a foul tackle or started running off with the ball in a different direction entirely from the goal; they just carried on, involving him just as much as anyone else in the game. And this isn't me saying, look how brilliantly they included him, mainstream is totally where Oscar needed to be, but it did make me smile to see him playing. It did ease my worries about the future a little because, for a few short moments, I'd looked on and seen how far he'd come. We still didn't know what the right or wrong decision was. We could put in the paperwork for a specialist placement and if we got a school, we could decide much closer to the time. But what I did know at this stage, is that we REALLY didn't want to get it wrong.

* * * *

In the Easter holidays, whilst Chris was away, I took the kids to a local play scheme. We'd been there loads of times as it's somewhere I felt I could take all three children on my own, also they loved it. It was safe, and no one (mentioning no names) could run off. The session was an hour and a half. Twenty minutes in, though, I realised that Oscar had had an accident.

Not sugar-coating it, it was an accident of epic proportions; I knew that I had to get Oscar into the toilet to change him ASAP. As I expected, he lost his sh**t (no pun intended) when I told him we had to leave the room and get cleaned up. He dropped to the floor and when I tried to hold his hand to help him up, he started shouting and flailing around. What was that again about people with DS always being 'SO happy'! Anyway, feeling people's stares and catching the eye of the odd person stood there watching, the general feeling I was getting from everyone was horror and disbelief. Members of staff stood and looked on too. When I eventually got him into the loo, his hysteria escalated to another level. I hadn't even had a chance to tell Alfie and Flo where I'd gone and, whilst I was sure they'd be fine, dealing with Oscar, his mess and wondering whether the other two were going to panic that I'd gone, I felt anxious. I had a spare pair of jeans for Oscar but no clean top (I told you it was epic), so I took the decision, even though we'd only been there for a few minutes, to get us all the hell out of there, pronto.

As I got us all back in the car, I felt emotional. Firstly, because of the way both Alfie and Flo had reacted. I'd told them that we were leaving minutes after we'd arrived there and I'd expected them to lose it, but instead they'd calmly said it was okay and walked out behind me. Whilst there may be times when things like this happen because of Oscar and they may feel disappointed or hard done by that they are missing out because of him, I really think in this instance they understood more than I'd previously given them credit for. I also felt emotional because I was annoyed at myself because I'd not only lost my temper with Oscar, but I'd been embarrassed. Something I'd vowed I would never be. I'd never wanted to apologise for my son and his behaviour, so I was cross with myself for feeling like that. But my main issue with all this and the reason I'd started to cry once I got home was that I couldn't believe that not one person, not a fellow mum nor even a member of staff in that entire place, had asked if they could do anything to help. No one asked if I needed anything or offered to keep an eye on Alfie and Flo for me. In true British style, they stood and watched or pretended it wasn't happening and, in that moment, I couldn't have felt more alone if I had tried.

And when I wrote about the experience online afterwards, most people said they'd like to think they would have helped. But a handful said they know they wouldn't have, for fear of me thinking that THEY thought I couldn't cope, or of making me cross. So, here's the thing. In my opinion (and I know I'm not speaking for every mother out there), if you ever see a mum of a little one struggling in the future, offer the help. I'm not saying I expected someone to clean my child's shit up, but perhaps someone checking to see if I had enough wipes or telling me they'd watch the other two, in that moment I know would have really helped me. When I've offered another mum a hand before and she hastily rebuffed my offer, I probably did feel a bit put out by her abrupt response, but I would far rather be on the receiving end of that than worry that I'd left her feeling helpless or like she'd wanted the world to swallow her up, like I had that day.

And on the back of that poo story, something that happened the following week restored my faith in humankind. . .

Picture the scene. We'd entered the zoo. The kids had been excited to see the meerkats except, on the way, they'd spotted the merry-go-round and had immediately asked to have a go. Persuading them that we could do so later, but first we should see some animals, my mum and I managed to head them off in the other direction to find our old friend Sergei. Except this merry-go-round was on the main thoroughfare, so we kept having to walk past it and every single time it was, 'Can we have a go nooooooooow?' Eventually we gave in and, feeling slightly harassed (what is it with vast open spaces, family attractions and three strong-willed offspring, all having an opinion on which direction they'd like to go in, that makes you want to pack up and go home minutes after arriving?), we paid for the three of them to go on. I'd asked the guy in the kiosk if I could stand with Oscar while it went round; however, I realised that all the horses had belts so, deciding he'd be fine, I got off before it started. As I was heading out of the exit, the man behind the kiosk called me over. Asking me what I was doing, I explained that Oz didn't need me after all. He smiled, then reached under his desk and pushed £2.50 towards me. 'Here,' he said, 'Go and get yourself a cup of tea.' Feeling puzzled, I asked what he meant – £2.50 had been the cost of one of the kid's rides so I realised he was essentially giving me one for free. Perhaps he'd seen just a few moments before Oscar sitting on the floor and me crouched down next to him because he'd seen the ice cream stand, had wanted one and I'd said no. Perhaps he'd seen the stand-off we'd had as he refused to move, and I refused to give in. Perhaps he'd simply thought, 'Blimey!

Look at her with her three kids trying to take back control of the situation.' I don't know. But his response was again, 'Go on, go and get yourself a cup of tea. You deserve it.'

I don't think I particularly deserved it any more than the next mum negotiating their way through the Easter holidays with their kids, but what I do know is that for a brief time, my faith in people and their kindness was restored.

After Easter, with the boys back at school, I went to empty Oscar's fruit pot and drink out of his school bag and found this.

Dear Oscar,

You are my best boy friend. You are so sweet and funny. I love you inside and out just by being you. I give you hugs everyday.

Love xxxxx

* * * *

The day had finally arrived. I had done all the training I could. Today was the day I was to run the London Marathon for a charity very close to my heart, the Down's Syndrome Association. I'd done every single training run on my own as I'd never wanted to put any pressure on myself to run at someone else's pace and here I was now, about to run 26.2 miles alone, but alongside some 40,000 other competitors. I had got a coach up to Greenwich with a local running club. A friend of mine who was a member of the club had said they wouldn't mind me grabbing a lift with them. I sat in silence listening to all their 'running chat' all the way to London. These guys weren't messing around; a lot of them would be trying for a PB, a personal best. I, at this point, would be happy just to make it round; I wasn't really thinking of speed. And I wasn't fast. In fact, at certain points I'm pretty sure I could have walked quicker on a normal day, but I ruddy well did it. Five hours and thirty minutes later, I'd finished. At the start, I'd met some of the others who were running for the same charity, and it was so lovely to see them all at the finish, where the DSA had put on food and drink for all of us. Chris and I had talked about the children coming to watch, but we'd decided it would be a bit too much for them, with all the crowds. A part of me had wanted Oscar there at the end; after all, I'd done this in honour of my biggest boy, but I gave him an extra-big squeeze when I saw him the following day, so happy that I had done this for him. I can honestly say that taking part in the London Marathon was both the hardest and the most brilliant thing I have ever done. I had so much support from my friends, family and even some people who'd followed me on my social media pages, which had helped to propel me round the course. I managed to raise, through the generosity of others, just over £7,500. A massive amount for the most wonderful and deserving charity.

Blog Comments

'I would say that the birth of any child is the beginning of a love story, but that the birth of a child with DS is the beginning of a love story with an extra-special sparkle. Expect there to be highs and lows, but that your heart will burst with love and pride.'

Claire Putland

'Be scared, but then do it anyway. Give your child a chance to see what other kids do so they want to do it too. Grit your teeth through the tough stuff because everything that is difficult to overcome will be more precious as it helps your child develop.

And hugs. All the hugs. Accept the hugs; you will need them and deserve them.'

Jayne Wallace

'I would tell myself you are making up all these terrible scenarios based on what? I thought we wouldn't bond. I thought we would never go on vacation again. I thought he wouldn't have a personality. So many worries based on nothing but my uninformed mind.'

Michelle Doran

17

Actual Big-boy PANTS!

The Royal Brompton respiratory team had referred Oscar to Guy's and St Thomas' Hospital as, although they knew that he had abnormal sleep patterns (his CO_2 dipped at night), they wondered if by speaking to a clinical psychologist who specialises in sleep it might flag up other reasons he had been so unsettled at night. The reflux medicine we'd been prescribed hadn't worked, which was frustrating, but at least it ruled out reflux as the cause of his trouble sleeping. To be honest, I hadn't been holding out that much hope, assuming they'd say that it was 'behavioural', which you often hear when it comes to anything to do with kids who happen to have DS. But this clinical psychologist was literally the kindest, loveliest man, who sat and listened to everything I had to say and gave me advice that gave me a teeny-tiny glimmer of hope that, with some changes, we might be able to at least make things a bit better.

A lot of what he spoke about was the environment Oz was sleeping in. Some of it felt like common sense, like the light level, the temperature and so on. But he also suggested we play pink noise (different from white noise) in the room. He suggested we use bergamot, an essential oil which releases a scent that tells the brain to associate it with sleep. We spoke about how sitting with him every night as he drifted off wouldn't be helping because when he wakes up he wants us still to be sitting there. He asked about Oscar's iron levels, which, the last time they'd been tested, had been low. He said that anyone with low ferritin levels is, of course, going to be restless at night-time. He said it was essential we got those levels up (Oscar had up until now refused the medicine he'd been prescribed, so shortly afterwards he started taking an iron supplement). The psychologist also said that there is a different type of melatonin to the one Oscar is on, not a tablet, but still slow-release. He described it as a small pellet that you can easily hide in food, but also that he should have his tonsils and adenoids properly checked, which we could do the following month, when he was going in for surgery on his ear.

The thing that gave me the most comfort, though, was that he didn't think it was behavioural because he'd been having the longest period of his sleep between 7 p.m. and 12 a.m. and that perhaps something was happening around midnight with regard to his breathing that had been waking him? It was a lot of information. Too much to change straight away, but we had options now and all any sleep-deprived mum wants is a little guidance, a little understanding and perhaps just a flicker of hope to hold onto.

It was six years ago to the day that Oscar had had open-heart surgery at the Royal Brompton Hospital, in London. I always talked about that day as having been the most horrific day of my life. And having previously felt that his unexpected diagnosis was my worst day, it was six years ago today that I realised that losing Oscar topped that, and just didn't bear thinking about. I remember hearing from a woman whose sister had needed heart surgery in the 1970s, but because this young woman had Down syndrome, she wasn't eligible. She spoke of how her father, through his passion and rage, had ended up pinning the doctor against the wall until he'd agreed to do the surgery. He eventually complied and the happy ending to this tale is that she lived to tell it. The anniversary of Oscar's surgery was always a poignant time for me, not only because we will always be so entirely grateful to the team who cared for him but also because it wasn't until 1976 that this operation was offered to those who happen to have DS. Up until that point, it was considered that their lives were seemingly of less value than yours or mine. If Oscar had been born forty years earlier, he too would have been refused the surgery.

* * * *

The kids stayed up a little later as we were on holiday in Mallorca. There was a live band playing and from the moment it started, Oscar stood up, took to the centre of the dance-floor, which had no one on it apart from him, and danced. He danced and danced, without a care in the world. Like no one was watching. Except, they were. A room full of people were watching my boy, literally having the time of his life. Without that heart surgery back in 2013 it's a given that Oscar wouldn't be here right now. Each year, on his 'heart anniversary', I always take some time to acknowledge the amazing NHS, the Royal Brompton and his surgeons. But this particular year, I spent some time recalling the story of the girl and her father who challenged that doctor and persuaded him that his daughter's life meant JUST as much as that of the next child. We owe him thanks for paving the way for so many children like ours, for without any of that, Oscar wouldn't be here, spreading a little happiness wherever he goes.

* * * *

I'd lost count of the number of times Oz had had surgery by now. This one was small fry compared with some of the operations he'd had in the past; he was only in theatre for forty minutes, the quickest yet. But he was now the proud owner of a titanium tube implant in his left ear, which apparently, in simple terms, is a more sophisticated grommet, which they were hoping would ultimately help his hearing. Like most things, he had taken it all in his stride. He used to cause such a fuss when it was time for the nurses to take his obs (observations – blood pressure, temperature, saturation levels for those not down with the medical lingo), but I'd noticed as time went by that very gradually he was becoming much less fearful.

There has been a lot of chat in the Down syndrome community about how some parents of those children and young adults who happen to have DS who are deemed not quite so able or who have a dual diagnosis (DS and autism), feel like their children aren't represented. The general feeling is that sometimes people give false hope to new parents and an unrealistic view of the challenges some families will face to the general public because not everyone's child turns out to be as 'able' as Oscar, for example. I'd also heard a few comments about Oscar being 'high-functioning' and it made me think about the way he was perceived, and if I do paint too 'perfect' a picture. There has been a lot in the media about the #wouldntchangeathing campaign. Whilst I love what the families behind it stood for, I had also openly said that whilst I wouldn't change Oscar for the world, there are a lot of things associated with him having Down syndrome that if I were able to, I would absolutely change for him, such as health-related issues, speech and communication delay etc.

It was looking more and more likely that Oscar would be moving from mainstream to a SEN placement when he made the transition into Year 3 and, if I'm honest, I was torn about whether I wanted to talk about it with others in our DS community. For some ridiculous reason I felt that if I admitted that that was the way we thought we were headed, that would mean we were admitting defeat. I'd been busy visiting an array of different SEN schools – both LAN (learning assisted needs, e.g. moderate learning needs) centres and SLD (severe learning difficulties) schools – to try to figure out where Oscar would best fit. It was a minefield. I was trying so desperately hard to resist the temptation to disregard a school because it had 'severe' in its title because it's just a word, right? It was just another label I could choose to be offended by, or not, and right now I was choosing to focus on what was best for my little man.

We'd been invited to London Zoo to a press event for the launch of their new children's play and discovery area, Animal Adventure. Before receiving the invitation, I had already booked and paid for Oscar to attend a play session at the charity for children who have additional needs, a session he attends two or three times during most school holidays because he loves it there. Reluctant to cancel that, I decided Alfie, Flo and I would go along without him. Having posted a series of InstaStories on my account, I then received a message from someone who followed me, saying: 'Didn't you feel bad sending Oscar to a play scheme today when you were taking the others to the zoo? I would.'

I wasn't upset or cross as I've learned over the years that for every one person who disagrees with something, there are a whole heap of others who agree, and this was, ultimately, just her opinion. I imagined the woman messaging me didn't have a child with additional needs herself. For if she had, I THINK (of course, I can't speak on behalf of all of us) she would understand that sometimes a few hours of respite for parents and siblings isn't necessarily a bad thing and is often very welcome. I will admit that Oscar probably would have loved a day out at London Zoo with the rest of us. But, truthfully, just for a few short hours, I was able to give my other two children the attention they so desperately crave and deserve. For a short time, I was able to relax and not be constantly pre-empting Oscar running off, or scanning the area for potential dangers. I wasn't asking Alfie to chase after his brother or for either him or Flo to stand still and not move while I hotfooted it after Oz myself. For a short while, I'll admit, I had been able to breathe.

And for the record, that isn't because I don't love spending time with Oscar the rest of the time. It isn't because I resent him or the life we have or that I really gave too much thought to how different it was with Oscar there or not (this was our 'normal'). So, I make no apology for leaving him behind that day, because not only could I say, hand on heart, that he was safe and happy where he was; I also know how important it is to give my other children the time they need too. I appreciate that by sharing our lives, I'm opening myself up to criticism. But to the woman who sent me that message, or to anyone else wondering why I'd do such a terrible thing, I'm hoping that's made things clearer. And truly, until any of us has walked for some time in someone else's shoes, none of us should be passing judgement on something we don't have first-hand experience of.

Some days I really feel like I'm on top of this parenting lark. Others? Like the time Oz decided to take off across Newbury Rugby Club's pitch, up the stairs of their clubhouse and into the building, where we were definitely not meant to be, it kind of felt like I was just about making it through the day.

We'd been on Day 2 of toilet training (I mean, this had been ongoing for quite some time, but this particular time I'd decided to go cold turkey with him and bite the bullet). It was apparently going to be the hottest day of the year so far, Chris had just turned off the water to sort out our leaky shower and Sainsbury's had just emailed to say that the ice lollies that were supposed to be included in my delivery, which I'd been expecting any minute, weren't available and there was no alternative. You'll be pleased to hear, though, that the carpet cleaner was included in my delivery.

Fast forward to two weeks later and we were getting there.

For some time, we – and the school – had been attempting to put him on the toilet and, if I'm honest, we weren't having much luck, or getting much co-operation, at all. Oscar had never shown any interest in wanting to sit on the toilet. He'd either get cross or seemed almost scared at the prospect. On occasion he would tell us that his nappy was wet or soiled but mostly it didn't seem to bother him that he was walking around with a full nappy.

I had joined a relatively new Facebook group, DSUK Going POTTY!, and had found loads of advice on there. Knowing that we had the summer holidays ahead of us, we went for it. We'd decided that initially Oz would be better on a potty, although we appreciated that there would be the issue of needing to transition him to the toilet next, but this was what we felt would be best for him. It meant that it was close by when he needed it and that helped, because when he needed to go there was (and sometimes still is!!!) a very short 'window'. We got him one that looked like a real toilet, which he seemed much more enthusiastic about sitting on. For the first three days, we didn't leave the house. We had an egg-timer that we set to ring every thirty minutes and Oscar eventually got that every time it rang it was 'wee wee time' (picture us singing this and making a huge fuss about the fact that it was all exciting). My mum very kindly took Alfie and Flo out a lot over those three days, but when they were around, they themselves thought it was brilliant when the timer went off and would shout 'wee wee time' – the team effort, I realised, helped to encourage Oscar. Initially, we were focused on getting him to 'try'. But I quickly realised that we could catch the odd wee on the potty. It also seemed that he had the capacity to hold it in for extended periods, sometimes for hours and hours. I also noticed that when he had a wee accident and I shouted, 'Stop,' he was able to stop the flow. We'd then run to the potty and he'd finish off on there.

There was lots of praise for every attempt to sit on the toilet, big cheers for successes on there, and I tried so hard not to make a big deal about the accidents (and there were LOTS). And, honestly, we saw big improvement in what was essentially a relatively short period of time. We started with incentives, for example, if you sit down and try you can have some sweeties or if you 'perform' you get a sticker, but we found quite quickly that we didn't need them, as I'm sure he'd grasped that I wasn't giving up on this and, 'FFS, Mum, I'll sit down and give it a go as you're clearly not dropping this,' had been his internal monologue. When we were at home there were significantly fewer accidents than when we were out and about, but I gauged he would get quite distracted when he was out somewhere. But when he was at home, he had mastered going when the timer went off, which I had now increased to every hour, or he would take himself. And, although he couldn't say the words, 'I need a wee,' he'd often come up to me, point to his willy, jiggle around on the spot and when I said, 'Do you need the toilet?' he would say yes and off we would run.

We even managed to use actual toilets out and about and he seemed much happier and more willing to sit on them. We had an incident in an M25 service station the other day, when he'd held his wee for over two hours so, having just made it to the loo, as I was about to sit him on it, it all became too much to bear and instead of anything going in the bowl, I was sprayed in the face and all over my clothes!!!!! I mean, let's face it, we've all been there when we've been so close, yet so far.

Anyway, amongst the DS community, there seemed to be two trains of thought on this:

1. You should wait until you feel your child is ready.
   or
2. Your child may never show signs of being ready, so you will literally have to 'train' them.

The advice now seems to be to start them as young as possible with sitting on the potty or toilet rather than waiting, to just go for it. In hindsight, perhaps we should have started Oscar when he was much younger, but I do feel strongly that you, as parents, must be ready to do it too. I waited until Alfie and Flo were a few months off three years old and they both got it within forty-eight hours.

With Oscar, we'd always known we were in it for the long haul. It was never going to be a quick fix like the other two. The first time he managed a poop in the toilet he walked away for a while, then went back of his own accord to finish off (sorry, TMI!). I can't tell you how much anti-bac I got through back then. I saw A LOT of bare bottom and willy. I spent my life savings on toilets, egg-timers, treats, car-seat protectors, Dry Like Me pads, travel potties, liners for travel potties and wipes – LOTS of wipes!!!! Our sofa was now covered in protective sheets and I may or may not have shouted at Chris yet again, because the poor guy really can't cope with poo but when it's all got a bit much for all involved, 'Did he really want to be changing this kid's nappies at twenty-five because I sure as hell didn't want that?' #relationshipgoals. It had taken years, but we were getting there.

We were going away on holiday later that week, so I'd been a little apprehensive about not wanting to go backwards. While I'm not saying it had been a walk in the park – walking around M&S Food Hall knowing Oz had a big old turd in his pants, was wearing shorts and at any given moment the offending turd could potentially make an appearance down his leg was a particularly low point – it hadn't been half as bad as I'd imagined it might be. With the benefit of hindsight, perhaps we should have tried properly before we did, but, as a very wise woman once told me, hindsight, much like poo at times, is an annoying pain in the arse.

We arrived home after two-and-a-half weeks away in beautiful Switzerland. It had been fab to get some sunshine, for the children to try new activities, but mostly for us all to be together. As a side note, I wouldn't advise going on holiday a few weeks after toilet training commences. Especially when you're staying in your in-laws immaculate chalet, as I had spent the best part of those two-and-a-half weeks braced with anti-bac and kitchen roll, just in case. (To be fair, Oscar had been an absolute star and had done so well.) And while it had been far from relaxing, having time away had given us the chance to really reconnect. I mean, it's amazing how much 1:1 time you spend with a person when you have a sneaky suspicion they're about to curl one out. In short, it had been lovely.

Pre-children, I don't think the word 'milestones' featured much in my life, yet when you have a child of your own, and particularly a child who perhaps struggles a little more to achieve said milestones, you can become dangerously consumed by when they'll reach the next one. I'm contacted a lot by parents of little ones asking me when Oscar first sat up, when he crawled and when he walked. And knowing that our kids, those who happen to have DS, all do things at their own pace, I try hard to reassure them that the kids will get there when they're ready. As I've said, before the summer, we'd attempted to toilet train Oscar several times. It was an ongoing project, with trips to the loo to at least 'try'. He'd watch Daddy pee, with us hoping that he'd suddenly feel this overwhelming urge to give it a go too, but honestly, without sounding harsh, Oscar couldn't have cared less. He had zero interest in sitting on the toilet; he was far too busy to entertain such a tedious task and, if I'm honest, I had visions of me bent over changing him and doing the walk out to the wheelie bin with a bag full of nasties for years to come.

But this September had been a momentous one. I'd sent Oscar back to school in pants. No nappies, no pull-ups, actual big-boy PANTS. And having been back a whole week now, in the entire time he'd been there, he'd had just one accident, one which had happened, incidentally, during the first twenty minutes of Day 1, when I imagine he was feeling a little wobbly – new class, new teacher etc.

And when Oscar had his heart check-up in London, we'd driven up and back, which with traffic was a good hour and half up and an hour and a half back and in that whole time, again. . . not one accident!!!! And this isn't about being a Braggy Brenda, because we all know that's not cool and often backfires, but when we're all at that stage and, let's face it, as SEN parents, we've all been there at one time or another, when you've lost all faith that they'll ever reach that next step, when you've pretty much given up all hope, they'll turn it around 360 degrees and show you just how bloody brilliant they are. I didn't doubt there'd be setbacks, but I was just so chuffing proud!!!

Blog Comments

'Gerard stopped wearing pads during the summer holiday before he started secondary school. We never forced the issue. He would use the toilet prior to this, usually before bed to get a routine but he was quite unpredictable. But we got there in the end. Now he's like a camel and I don't know where he stores it as he can go hours. We still support him in the bathroom, but I am so glad we can leave the house without a big changing bag.'

Bernadette Andrea

'Consistency and routine helped Tobi. Lots of spare joggers and pants. We encouraged Tobi to go regularly, and school were very supportive too. Tobi was toilet trained by six, day/night and although he wipes himself now, I do need to still help him and he's now eleven.'

Lisa Ellis Easthop

'We tried Noah on the potty in the morning just after his first birthday and very quickly he started reliably doing a wee and poo on the potty first thing in the morning. He suffers from constipation due to having Gaviscon in his feeds and we found the position on the potty really helped him. We are gradually building more potty time in during the day.'

Claire Oakley

18

A Duck, Paddling For Dear Life

'Because every picture tells a story'
Unknown

A few years ago, the prospect of half-term approaching would have filled me with horror. Having spent a while now standing at the school gates, listening to #Mumchat, I have a confession to make. When mums say things like, 'I can't wait till the kids break up for half-term,' or, 'It's going to be so nice to have them at home with me,' although I may have looked like I was agreeing with them, the voice inside my head was thinking, 'ARE YOU CRAZY!?'

It was totally my fault for having three children so close together and I appreciate I have only myself to blame (well, Chris may have had a teeny part in all this too), but I was a much better mum when I had one, or a maximum of two, at a time because, when I had all three, it usually all turned to s**t!! Taking all three out to any sort of overcrowded public attraction at the same time could at times back then be problematical. They all wanted to do their own thing and as much as I would have loved to have let them, the times I did, well, it resulted in thinking I'd lost one or more of them, causing major heart palpitations. That has usually been remedied with a large glass of Sauv Blanc at the end of the day, declaring to Chris, 'Well, I'm a dick for even thinking THAT was a good idea.'

But I've actually now realised that I don't get that panicky feeling as much. I mean, okay, while we'd been at a pumpkin farm, Oscar had managed to cause a minor scene because when repeatedly told by staff members not to run along the hay bales, he'd completely ignored them and carried on. But focusing on the positive, he'd not been running off, right? I liked hanging out with the children now. They really made me laugh. Flo, with a side order of sass. Alfie, because he teaches me random facts most days – 'Did you know that an octopus has nine brains and three hearts, Mummy?' 'Ummmmm, no, Alfie, I didn't know any of that.' And Oz, being a man of few words, had recently mastered 'ssshhhhing' me when he wanted me to stop singing so loudly. I suppose they'd all grown up. And, whilst a few years ago, I had been struggling to see through the fog, now? I found myself quite enjoying spending time with them.

Oscar had been invited to the birthday party of one of his friends. This little boy had chosen six friends and Oscar had been one of those six. The party had the theme of a sports day of sorts and they played a series of games – cricket, welly wanging, a treasure hunt, dodgeball and a football match. It had been right up Oscar's street and he'd loved every minute of it. When it came to the football game, I was standing quite some distance from where the boys were playing. Although I was talking to the other parents there, I always had one eye on Oscar, not because I thought he would run off (the likelihood of that was slim because nothing can usually tear him away from a football these days), but knowing he had previous, I knew I could never really afford not to be watching. . . just in case. As I watched, I saw one of the boys tackle another boy, who fell to the ground. He'd obviously been hurt and while the rest of the group seemed oblivious to this (unwavering in their quest to get that goal), Oscar noticed the boy on the floor and ran over to him to help him up. I then watched as he appeared to lean in towards him (I assumed to give him some sort of nod of encouragement) and then stand momentarily rubbing his back. Within a few seconds the hurt boy was seemingly fine, gave Oscar a smile and off he went in pursuit of the ball. It was a small act. One of those blink-and-you-miss-it moments. And perhaps to anyone else it wouldn't have been that big a deal at all. But watching Oz and that little act of kindness was the sweetest moment.

* * * *

Oscar and I had taken the train in to London as he had a casting. We got on the Tube, walked to the casting, had a little chat with the woman in charge, had his photos taken and returned home. Throughout the morning he behaved beautifully. He told me when he needed the toilet, didn't run off and was generally stress-free to be around. Don't get me wrong, there were still days when he could run rings around me. Like on the mornings he felt the incessant need to be in front of the person walking in front of us on the school run, meaning that in a busy village with streams of people walking to school, we had to essentially skip, jog and run all the way there, with Alfie and Flo in tow. There were days when I would find myself thinking, 'Other parents of seven-year-olds have far surpassed this stage, yet here I am, still chasing my child up the high street.' But then there are moments, like this one in London or at the football game, when I realise how fast time flies and, just like that, you're being reminded of acts of kindness and the impact they can have on others.

That November, Oscar attended his first Chelsea Foundation DS Active Session. The sessions took place on a monthly basis at Chelsea's training ground in Cobham and to say it was a success would be an understatement – OSCAR ABSOLUTELY LOVED IT! He had been in a group with four other children his age, all of whom had Down syndrome themselves, and they had two coaches leading them. Chris had taken him along, but he was sending me regular text updates throughout, the consensus being that Oscar was doing well and that Chris thought he had pretty good hand-eye co-ordination. Chris said the coaches had been kind, patient and took the time to really get to know each child, working out quickly who needed extra guidance at times. Oscar had loved playing football from a really young age and would always be the first to jump in on a game if anyone was playing in our local park, but up until now, because local groups hadn't seemed open to him joining, apart from kick-abouts in the garden at home, he hadn't really had the chance to give the sport a proper go. Anyway, the day after he'd trained with Chelsea Football Club and before his bath, Oscar saw that I was packing his backpack (ready for school the next day). He ran straight over to me, signed 'football' and started jumping up and down, excited at the prospect of heading off to training again. When I broke it to him that he wasn't going to football, he stood there in front of me and burst into tears. He was devastated not to be going. Any chance he got he'd been asking to see the photos Daddy had sent me on my phone of him playing. And now I had the job of breaking it to him that the next sessions weren't for a whole month.

* * * *

It's silly, really. It was just a school photo, after all. Flo had started at the boys' school back in the September and just before Christmas we'd received a photograph from the school, of all three of them together in a shot. I'd loved it. They were all in the same green uniform, all smiling at the camera: it was the classic sibling school photograph. As time rolls on for other groups of siblings, a photo like this one will be replaced each year as they move up through the year groups and continue their time in school together. But for me, the photo meant so much more as this would almost certainly be the first and last photo of this kind because this academic year was the first and last time Oscar, Alfie and Flo would all be at the same school.

We were to find out later that week if Oscar had got a provisional place at our named SEN school from September 2020 and, whilst I knew in my heart, that this was the right decision for Oscar, there was something playing out in all of this that felt like a grief of sorts. I guess it was about letting go of the path I had thought we would be taking and finding a different way. I was treasuring every second of having all three of them all together in one place that year. From time to time, they'd tell me they'd 'found' each other in the playground, how they'd seen one another in reflections (assembly) or how they'd helped each other to the office when one of them had fallen over. And I wasn't sure if everyone would understand, that when I looked at that photo, it represented both happiness and pride that they'd had this time together at school; but also that it was tinged with just a tiny bit of sadness too.

The previous year at the nativity play, Oz had taken centre stage and danced his little heart out, as I sat silently weeping. The tears had mostly been because I'd been so proud of him. I'd also been crying with laughter, at the enthusiasm, at his dance moves and I suppose because he had adopted the mantra of 'Dance like nobody's watching' and gone for it. This year, he'd had two opportunities to show us all what he was made of. The morning show that I watched and then the afternoon one that Chris had rushed all the way back from Birmingham for. Except both times, when it came to his dance, he remained seated and wouldn't get up. While the other children in his group tried to encourage him, whispering to him to come and dance, he'd sat pretending he hadn't heard them. When his TA, who'd been sitting a short distance away, crawled on her hands and knees to reach him and gave him what I can only imagine were some words of encouragement, he'd pretended she wasn't there and turned his head away. In the second show, having used some with him already, they'd gone to the trouble of printing out more visual cues, to show him what was coming next, only to be met with a vigorous shake of the head and a refusal to move, commonly known in this house, as 'sit and protest'. Aside from standing up to attempt to sing and sign the songs they'd practised (I say this loosely, in that sometimes, whilst the entire school were stood there using Makaton, he didn't even bother doing that), for the most part Oscar outright refused to do his bit in the school nativity play this year. So, just in case any of you were under the illusion that Oscar performs on demand, I can confirm that that is very much a lie. This kid knows his own mind and when he's not feeling something, there can be no swaying him from his chosen course of action, or inaction. The silver lining in all this is that Alfie and Flo smashed it. So, you know, rough with the smooth.

* * * *

I'd overheard something that probably wasn't meant for my ears. It was silly, really, because I know kids often say things without thinking but somehow this comment, a throwaway comment that they probably haven't given much thought to since, I bet, has stayed with me. We were walking down the street, Oscar jogging a little in front of me and between us was a little boy of six or seven walking with his mum. He'd obviously seen Oscar dart past them both and in a very loud voice exclaimed, 'That's Oscar. He's really naughty, Mummy.' Initially, the woman didn't say a word, I'm guessing because she knew I was almost directly behind them, only her silence meant he repeated it again, in a much louder voice. I'm not sure what she said as a response as she was obviously speaking a lot more quietly, but I'm guessing she was inwardly cringing at how this was all unfolding, just as much as I was walking behind them both. It didn't stop there, though, as he then launched into something about Oscar always shouting and how he hit someone once before.

I felt for the woman. Mostly because I could feel her squirming as I probably would have done had it been one of my children. It wasn't the time nor the place to talk to this little boy and explain why Oscar is loud sometimes, when everyone is supposed to be being quiet. Neither was it the right time to talk to him about why sometimes Oscar might be a bit rougher than the next child, due to a need to seek sensory stimulation, an inability to communicate verbally and feeling frustrated, but I really hoped that the next time this woman and her son had a quiet moment together that she would say to him that Oscar didn't mean to be 'naughty', that he wasn't badly behaved or disobedient, that there were just some times when he finds things a little harder to learn or to understand what's expected of him.

Out of all the children that we meet, whether in his school, in the community, friends, friends of friends or family, MOST of them get it. Most of them are accepting and understanding of Oscar and the little things he does. But occasionally, when you come across a little boy like this one, even though you don't blame him for what he says – you don't even blame the parents in that moment because we can't control everything that comes out of our children's mouths, you just hope they can educate them gently about accepting people who might be a little different from them – it still feels like you've somehow been punched in the stomach every single time. And not because you're being overly sensitive, but because if you ask any parent of a child with SEN all they want for their child is for them to be accepted and understood in society and the fear that they might not be is heart-breaking.

There is only seventeen months between Oscar and his little brother Alfie, but as time went on, Alfie far surpassed Oscar in most areas. It was tough on Alfie because in my mind, I'd put pressure on him to be the sensible one and I've always said that in a lot of ways he had to grow up just that bit faster. Alfie was the one who always had Oscar's back though. He was the one who, if we'd been in the park and another child had squared up to Oz, Alfie would step in and defend him, even if Oscar had been the one in the wrong. He'd shadow him as we walked to and from school each day, making sure he didn't step out into the road and he'd look after Flo for me if Oz had decided to do one of his 'sit and protests' and I couldn't get him to budge. He put up with a lot sometimes, but he just got it. He understood and, without any prompting or persuasion, he was his big brother's fiercest protector.

One day, on the way to school, Oscar got caught short and had a little accident. I knew he hadn't gone before we'd left home, an error on my part. He had told me he needed to go half-way up the road, but obviously with the walking fast and the cold wind. Eeeeek! Assessing we were closer to the school than home, I decided to head there to get him changed but as we were walking along, Alfie and Flo, who were just a few steps behind us, shared an exchange, that in the midst of me feeling super stressed out, melted my heart.

Alfie: Flo, we can't tell anyone that Oscar's wet his pants.

Flo: Why?

Alfie: Because everyone might laugh at him.

[Pause]

Alfie: I know, we'll just tell them that he splashed in a puddle. Yes, that's what we'll say, okay?

Flo: [Gasp] But that's a LIE, Alfie!

I mean, I know morally and ethically Flo was obviously right and this could have been an opportune time to talk to them about the importance of telling the truth, but I just loved Alfie's need to protect Oscar, probably himself too, of course, as who wants to be pissypants's brother? But it was just gorgeous and made my day.

* * * *

It had been a long wait for us, but we'd just found out that the school we'd named as our first choice for Oscar's transition into Year 3 had been agreed. Chris and I had spent a great deal of time looking at different types of schools in our area, some mainstream, others mainstream with a unit attached. We'd looked at different types of SEN settings, so we felt fully equipped to make a decision based on what we'd seen. And we'd made the decision to go with a SEN setting for children with learning and additional needs (LAN). Having spent the last few days anxiously scrolling forums and Facebook groups, seeing that some people had heard and others hadn't, I understood there were still several hundred children in Surrey who were yet to be placed in schools. The SEND admissions team, as I understood it, had been under a huge amount of pressure trying to finalise things. I also knew that there were still thousands of children every year excluded from schools because there just wasn't the appropriate school available for them. Knowing that we had a place for Oscar meant we had a renewed faith and hope that finally he'd be in a school where he could reach his full potential. The village school had been great for a while, but he had been coasting along for some time now and progress seemed to have slowed right down. It felt like a giant leap but one both he and we were excited about.

I'd decided that the February half-term wasn't my favourite. It was wet, cold and there was a limit to what you could do. Anything that was play-based inside was overcrowded, loud and essentially hell on earth, right? So, I concluded that I much preferred spring and summer when you could have the back doors wide open, the kids could run in and out and there wasn't any mud, just trampolines, slides and paddling-pool fun.

The thing was Oscar was so capable physically and could often outrun even the fastest kids, but taking him to any sort of indoor play scheme was sometimes just too overwhelming, mostly for me. On the Monday, we'd gone to a local role-play centre, but while parents of typical children his age and younger sat and enjoyed a cuppa, I tended to be just a couple of steps behind Oz – you get it now – just in case. It wouldn't ever be anything major – a nudge in the back to push another child down a slide; the snatching of a toy because he'd wanted to play with it and he simply didn't have the verbal communication skills to ask them nicely. Finding another child's pair of shoes, putting them on and walking away wearing them. You get the picture.

Over the years, I've had a lot of comments from friends and family telling me they thought we did a lot and, whilst I agree up to a point, I'll let you in on a little secret: I wasn't always enjoying it. I did it because I didn't want to stay at home all the time and I wanted my kids to have fun. But just so you're aware, although I may have looked like a swan gliding across the water holding it all together, underneath it all, I was a duck, paddling for dear life, just to get to shore.

Blog Comments

'My son is in Year 6 in a MS [mainstream] school and his school has been amazing, fully inclusive, they listen to me and my concerns and adapt to suit Elliot. One teacher even set up an after-school signing choir so other children could learn to sign and Elliot would be included in a school club.

He gets on well with everyone in his class and they are very supportive of him and help when he is struggling. He learns the same subjects as them but the work is adapted to his level so he can participate in all lessons. He has a close group of friends (mainly girls) that he's had from reception to now in Year 6.'

Emma Costello

'At twenty, Adam and his two friends randomly ring each other to check in on one another. It's often just to say hi (even though they've only been with each other at college an hour before) or to tell each other something obscure. It's amusing listening to them.'

Nicky Royalle Leggitt

'Now that Oliver has been in his SEN school for nearly ten years his friends continue outside the classroom. We meet up for bowling and walks during holidays and he also does basketball, football x 2 and cricket outside of school with his school friends.'

Ann Marie Funk

19

Nineteen Lessons From Home-schooling

'When everything seems to be going against you,
remember that the airplane takes off against
the wind, not with it'

Henry Ford

We'd had an appointment with Oscar's ENT consultant to
discuss the next steps as far as his hearing was concerned.
The situation currently was that Oscar's hearing had
deteriorated again; he had moderate hearing loss. The
titanium implants he had had operations to insert hadn't
worked. We could have gone down the route of having
further surgery, but the trouble was, the more surgery he
had on his ears, the more likely it was to cause further
damage or scar tissue, which could make everything
worse. We knew that people with DS have low muscle
tone (hypotonia), which affects the opening and closing
of the eustachian tube. The negative pressure builds up
in the middle ear, which then leads to fluid retention,
meaning that even if we did go ahead with surgery, there
was a likelihood it wouldn't work or, if it did, it wouldn't
last. So, we started talking about him potentially needing

hearing aids again. It was a topic that had come up once or twice over the years, but each time we thought we'd proceed, his hearing would get better. He'd had a BAHA (bone-conducted hearing aid on a headband) when he was around two to three-and-a-half years old, but he wasn't that great at tolerating it, which is why we'd opted for grommets (and then all the underlying cholesteatoma ear issues were revealed). We were hoping that this time, with Oscar being that little bit older, that if he realised they'd help, he would be more receptive to over-the-ear hearing aids.

Even though I'd known this was a possibility and was looking more and more likely, I couldn't help but feel a little sad about it all. I knew I was being ridiculous because if they helped, it would be great. But I guess it was that feeling of it being another hurdle again. Perhaps also, this was more about me internalising that this wasn't what I'd wanted for him again. Like the time he'd had to wear 'special boots' – it wasn't what I'd wanted for him then either. Like the time also I'd realised he wouldn't cope in a mainstream sports club without support. That wasn't what I'd wanted for him either. And the time we came to the realisation that mainstream school was too much for him; that really wasn't what I'd wanted for him, ever. Being a SEN parent is a constant battle in your head. You want them to be the one that defies the odds and, despite having DS, proves everyone wrong by being brilliant. But equally you don't want to put an expectation on them to be anything but their brilliant self, whatever that might look like. I regularly listen to so many new parents tell me that their baby is keeping up with their peers as far as milestones go and I can hear how they're holding onto that hope. I was that parent:

the one who'd hoped life would be easy for Oscar and that he'd sail through. Except I've learnt that there are twists and turns and ups and downs along the way and many a bump in the road.

Around January or February in 2020 there'd been talk in the media of a new virus, Covid-19, that was likely to spread. I didn't think too much of it at the time, completely naive as to what was about to happen and the impact this would have on the whole world. But, in March 2020, when we had learned more about the effects of the virus and the impact it was having, particularly on the vulnerable, with a national lockdown looming, Chris and I took matters into our own hands.

After much thought and discussion and with my anxiety levels elevated to new heights, we'd decided to pull all three of our kids out of school. The previous week, we'd met with Oscar's cardiac consultant, who had initially put our minds at rest that Oscar was a strong little boy, hadn't had any chest infections for several years and told us that if she were us, she would take comfort knowing that the viral infections he had had over the winter months he'd fought and hadn't needed any hospital admissions. A new statement was then released by Alder Hey Hospital, who are in charge of paediatric cardiac services, with updated guidelines regarding pulmonary hypertension, which Oscar had had in the past. That sealed the deal for us, and we decided we just couldn't risk him being in school with so many other children.

None of us had any symptoms of Covid-19, but it would have been counter-productive to keep Alfie and Flo in school because of the chance they'd bring home bugs and pass them on. So, we found ourselves locked down for the foreseeable future.

That first day, we managed to get out. (Whenever we could, we would, because three kids inside all day long was honestly my worst nightmare.) I hadn't planned a thing, but managed to wing a scavenger hunt in the woods, phonics, crafts, handwriting practice and 'PE' (e.g. swing-ball in the garden) and we'd got through it. I'm not sure the kids learned that much. Their initial reaction when I said I was going to be their teacher was to laugh, but come 3 p.m. I was the one reminding them that, technically, school would have been over by now and that it was okay for us all to chill out and watch a bit of telly (mainly because I was knackered). So, whilst we all got ten out of ten for enthusiasm, I'm certain I may have peaked too soon, as who the hell could keep up that sort of pace?

None of us knew at this point just how long we would 'stay home'. I think in my head I'd imagined it would be a few weeks and then we'd get back to normal, but here I am writing this, almost two years on, and Covid is still here, we're still being asked to isolate if we have it and it's still a big old shitshow. Okay, yes, we might be out of lockdown, but with the newest variant Omicron, infection rates are rising again despite so many people being vaccinated and boosted, so whilst I hope there won't be another full lockdown, there's every chance school bubbles could shut left, right and centre.

Anyway, back to March 2020. I should mention that despite thinking I'd had a lot, snacks were now dwindling. I recall asking Flo at 9.30 a.m. if she would have had that many snacks before this time at school? And I can't tell you how many packets of Steak McCoy's Oz devoured that first month, so forget a national shortage of toilet roll, we'd been on a hunt for more McCoy's.

When I think back to the days of 'home-schooling' it honestly sends me into a PTSD-like state. It wasn't something I'd ever envisioned being able to cope with – being home with three small children, but we got through it. Just. And in between the hiding in the loo (me) and shouting at Chris that he was lucky, as he got to escape to his man-shed each day and not get involved with split digraphs or number lines, I can look back now and realise, perhaps the kids and I learnt a little after all. . .

1. I think we were all in agreement that an episode of *Maddie's Do You Know?* was as good as a science lesson.

2. NO ONE in our house flushed the loo other than me.

3. Although Oz looked fully engaged in activities for short spaces of time, the reality was he couldn't have given fewer f**ks about how many Cheerios he'd managed to place on the toothpicks or counting to twenty.

4. At eighteen I'd had two options: to become a professional dancer or to train as a primary school teacher. I can confirm that I'd made the right choice for me.

5. What I'd saved in general life expenditure, it seemed I was now spending, tenfold, on Amazon prime/ Hobbycraft. #resources

6. Class Zoom chats were cute in theory, but it was unlikely you'd hear the kids over one another.

7. While you might think setting up an obstacle course in the garden will cover gross motor skills and a bit of maths ('Whose time was greater than, whose time was less than etc.'), it would almost certainly result in tears. #alfiealwayswins

8. However many snacks you think you've got in the cupboard, there are never enough (and labelled baskets with children's names on them only work for those whose kids haven't worked out how to unlock cupboards, or whose kids follow rules).

9. Disney+ subscription. #giftfromgod

10. Oscar getting hold of a harmonica whilst being locked down in a house was torture.

11. Although Joe Wicks was doing amazing things for the nation, we needed music, Joe!

12. I'd never cared for him much before then, but I was living for Boris's 5 p.m. updates (not so much by January 2022).

13. I'd always thought we'd been generous with our TA gifts at Christmas/end of year. . . but, in reference to point 3 above, we may need to reassess. #luxuryspabreakrequired

14. It was surprising what random dinners you could come up with. One evening? Southern fried chicken and cheesy leeks. #foodrationing

15. One day, whilst helping Alfie with his learning, I had to Google 'rectangular prism' (please refer to point 4).

16. Printer ink runs out fast.

17. Threatening (never encouraged, of course) to call Miss <insert teacher name here> used to work on my kids, but had now lost its impact because they knew there was no likelihood of seeing them any time soon.

18. Despite all this, it was rather lovely spending time with one another.

19. I had never been more grateful for the tireless work that health-care professionals, the emergency services, other key workers and shop assistants were all doing to

make things easier for those of us who'd been at home. I learnt that they are all incredible.

I imagine most people were feeling up and down, in survival mode and navigating the best way to get through each day. Parents were struggling with the new set-up everywhere, but perhaps more so, those who had children with additional needs.

Every morning Oscar would ask me (signing) if he was going to school. When I'd reply with, 'No, not today,' he'd always look puzzled, like he was trying to figure it all out. Alfie and Flo were really enjoying the fact that their teachers were setting them their learning each day. In the same way that I did, I think they liked the structure, but getting Oscar to sit for any extended period to concentrate on his learning was tough. While the other two liked me to be on hand to help them with their work, Oscar absolutely needed me with him to help him stay on task, so it felt like I was being pulled every which way.

Oscar's sleep has always been up and down. Even if he managed to sleep an entire night, which was rare – he normally wakes two to three times – he's always up around 5 a.m., sometimes earlier, meaning that that was when our day started together. And, without the respite of school, the day was long. He is a very physical little boy too. It isn't a constant thing, in that we do have periods of calm when he'll sit and play or watch his iPad, but a lot of the time Oscar was home, he had this incessant need to be on the go. What's confusing to those who don't know is that this is a sensory thing for Oscar. The jumping on the trampoline, the climbing on the slide, the scooting at speed – he is just trying to self-regulate and it became more obvious to me being at home with him so much just how much he needs that. And because we couldn't get out as we might have done on a normal day, we couldn't go to the playground to burn off some steam. He needed to be watched. All day. And it was exhausting.

What I will say, though, is that he was happy. While lots of children with additional needs weren't coping at all well with being out of routine, Oscar seemed to be enjoying being at home with his brother and sister. Lots of children would be struggling with anxiety and parents would be on edge about how they were going to cope with this in the longer term, but while we had our moments, mostly we were doing okay. When all this started, I decided not to put too much pressure on myself. Although I could give it a go, I wasn't and was never going to be, Oscar's teacher. I was there to make him feel safe and loved and I could do that bit, no problem. I forgave myself in advance for the fact that there'd be times that Alfie and Flo wouldn't have my full attention because Oscar often took me away from them. But I'd decided that the benchmark for how we were doing would be whether the kids and I were still smiling at the end of each day. And we had been. Mostly.

I knew there was an abundance of parents out there who'd been worrying about how they were going to get through every day. Those parents whose respite had been taken away, whether that be school, after-school activities and clubs or PA (personal assistant) hours and I knew it had been tough. There were those who couldn't take their kids to their local park because it was closed and that, during lockdown, had felt huge. There were those kids who were lashing out in frustration because they could not understand why they couldn't do all the things they'd done before. It was relentless for all, but a little more so for those families with kids who'd found things just that bit harder to comprehend.

In the weeks and months that followed, at least there was never a dull moment. On one particular day, Oscar managed to get a bead from the craft-box stuck up his nose (you'll know this isn't the first time this sort of thing has happened to him). I was once called to school to help retrieve a bead he'd managed to lodge up his nose and another time, as we were driving along, he had stuffed a mint tic tac up his nostril when I wasn't looking. He tapped me on the shoulder and pointed up there to let me know. Thankfully, by this time, we'd mastered the art of squeezing the bead-free nostril and blowing down through our noses to shoot the now snot-covered bead out.

Oscar also regularly managed to get into Flo's room and would chuck her duvet, pillows, drawers of clothes and numerous cuddly toys over the bannister and into the hallway, mostly when I was on the phone to a professional, calling up to see how he was getting on.

Then there was the time he found the grass seed Chris had ordered online. He'd opened a bag of it up and emptied the entire contents all over the floor. There was also the time he'd found the biscuits we'd made the day before and eaten the entire plate.

I mean, he hadn't tried to scale the garden fence for a while at this point, so, you know, small wins.

But amongst the 'never a dull moment' and 'you gotta laugh or you'll cry' times, there were a few times when I did just about lose it.

Alfie had been waiting for me to listen to him read, except I'd been called away to Oscar. When I returned, because I was so worked up and because by this stage Alfie had lost interest and didn't want to sit with me any more, I got cross. I shouted at him. He shouted back. So I shouted some more. And then, when he'd gone quiet, I told him that all his friends were at home doing THEIR learning with their parents and, knowing that he'd be mortified if he did, I asked him if he wanted to go down a reading band when he got back to school because that's what would happen if he didn't bother to practise reading.

I was an arsehole. I made him cry. Then I cried because that's what I did when I got frustrated, but also because I recognised that I'd lost control. The thing I realised with my kids, though, is that they didn't ever hold grudges. Not in the way Chris and I did when we had an argument; we could go hours without so much as looking at one another. No, when they know you're disappointed, all they want is for you not to be disappointed any more. They just want you to be happy again and to make it all better.

A few minutes later, I felt a kiss on my arm. It was Alfie.

We had a chat. I said I was sorry for getting cross. He said he was sorry he didn't want to do his 'learning'. So I sacked off trying to achieve anything with them that day and instead we had a little dance in the kitchen. There are some days when you really kid yourself into thinking you're nailing it. Other days, you just about get by. And then there are days when you find yourself sitting, having a little cry to yourself, because it's all got a bit too much. I knew I wasn't alone back then, in that I knew there were hundreds of thousands of us, if not more, feeling overwhelmed. Tomorrow was a new day.

Blog Comments

'My four-year-old daughter has DS and I have a nearly seven-year-old son. We have only in the last year discussed extra chromosomes with my son as we just assumed he knew as we have never not talked about it around him. However, he was oblivious. At least now when a peer asks why his little sister isn't doing the same as an age-matched sibling he can tell them. They've always got along well but recently they really play together more. My son looks out for his sister and helps her with things. They also fight, box and wrestle and I'm not sure who is the bad influence.'

Louise Kennedy

'We had three typical children, fourth pregnancy was planned, and we had Adam who was diagnosed with DS postnatally. We went on to have a little "surprise" baby number five who like his siblings, didn't have DS. Adam's siblings adore him. They take so much time to help him, they are always on hand to offer him whatever it is he wants. His younger brother and him have the closest bond. I do worry that if anything happens to me in the future, if they'd feel obliged to help care for him. But I don't think they would consider it an obligation – I believe they would feel it was a privilege to have him in their life and be able to support him and help him grow.'

Nikki Jennifer

'I'm both a sibling to my brother who has DS and a mum to my child who has DS. The best things about being a sibling to a person who has DS is that you do all things ferociously with your sibling. You love ferociously, play ferociously, fight ferociously and defend them ferociously!'

Ruth Hartnett Carr

20

'Thank You For Always Seeing Oscar First'

On the advice of Oscar's occupational therapist, I thought we'd give mark-making in shaving foam a go. Oscar had been working hard on trying to write his name – we'd nailed an O but hadn't got much further yet. The thinking behind sensory play is that your child can develop the feel and technique for forming different letters and numbers without the stress of having to control a pencil or crayon. Initially, we tried using little toy cars to make straight lines. We then tried curvy lines and zigzags, using straws. But honestly, as activities go, it wasn't THAT successful. Before I'd had kids, I had had visions of me being one of those 'craft' mums, who'd pull activities out of cereal boxes and paper bags. But I just don't think that'll ever be me. I guess with the shaving-foam exercise the target we did manage to tick off was having fun. I'll take that.

When we did manage an activity successfully, like the time I saved a shedload of eggshells, wrote numbers on them and got the kids to answer sums by smashing them, it was almost always balanced out with some times you'd rather forget. Like the day I spent trying to discourage Alfie from watching *Shark Attacks* on YouTube because at this stage he was having nightmares. All whilst stuffing my face with sugar because Oz had had an 'at home sleep study' done the previous night and I had been up most of the night trying to get the sensors, probes and nasal cannula to stay on him. Intercepting Oscar's latest game – throwing toys, kitchen utensils and items of clothing (remembering the time my pants went missing) over the garden fence – was up there as a personal lockdown highlight. Not.

We did have a little detour from the lockdown norm one morning, in that we'd taken Oscar to St George's Hospital for what we thought was going to be emergency surgery. Long story short, Oscar had an abscess on his bottom, just below his coccyx (we think caused by either a bite or cut that had got infected with bacteria) and when we'd gone up to A&E the night before because it was looking nasty, they had thought it needed draining. Oscar had been in quite a bit of discomfort and hadn't been himself, but he was still smiling, even if sitting down was posing a bit of a problem. Anyway, it turned out that when we got to the hospital, the surgeon decided not to operate and to wait to see how it looked once the antibiotics had kicked in. We were told to head back up there on the Monday to reassess, so were keeping our fingers crossed for no surgery.

Around this time, someone left a comment on a social media post of mine, from two years ago, which read, 'I had the NIPT testing done and found out we were having a boy. But also found out he's got a 91% chance of having Down syndrome so now instead of planning a gender reveal party, we're now planning an abortion.'

I often wonder why someone would write something on a post from years beforehand and I can only guess that they either search the hashtags (in this case #prenataltesting) or have spent some time scrolling through my pictures and posts to find something that resonates with them.

My first reaction when I read this was that it hurt. No matter how many times I'd told myself I was pro-choice (and believe me, I am, as in my opinion, every woman has the right to choose) comments like these always felt personal, for she was essentially saying, 'I don't want a child like yours.'

And I get that. I get what she thinks she sees. She sees that bringing a child like Oscar into the world means there'll be challenges. She sees the part about it not being easy and how some days, no matter how much I love him so completely and with my whole heart, she sees the not-quite-so-amazing things that come with having a child like him. I wonder if because I'm so open with my thoughts, in her mind it's okay to be open about her actions right back. I often wonder, though, when people contact me saying they're contemplating having, or have had, a termination because of DS, if it would be better left unsaid. To someone like ME at least. Someone who has a child they didn't initially want and still struggle sometimes with having?

But then I really think about it and try to figure out why it is people feel the need to share. Why they feel the need to write a comment like that one, on what's very apparently a page advocating for DS. And I can only conclude it's about THEM, more than it is about us and our life with Oscar.

Perhaps by stating it for all to see, it's about feeling better once it's written down. (I know I always feel better when I've got something off my chest). Maybe it's about acceptance. Maybe they're seeking my/our approval? Maybe they're trying to spark a reaction? Trying to goad me to get cross with them, so they can fight their corner and tell me all the reasons why they're right. To make them feel better perhaps.

A while ago, another woman contacted me who said she was contemplating an abortion because the baby she was carrying had DS. Her partner and her family were all trying to persuade her to have her child and while I tried my best to tell her all the wonderful things about having Oscar, she went quiet, and I never heard from her again. I knew what she'd done. I share our lives on my social media pages and books for those people interested enough to see that we're good. That despite the challenges, despite all of them, we're doing okay. Ultimately, I can't control what others think. Perhaps if the women who'd made those choices had stuck around long enough, they might have changed their minds. I don't know. What I do know is that in all the years I've been doing this, we have changed so many people's perceptions and, genuinely, I wish them only happiness.

That September, Oscar was moving to a specialist placement at a local SEN school. We hadn't expected that there'd be any settling-in sessions (because, you know, national pandemic and all that) but in June we'd had a call, asking if Oscar would like to go in and meet his new teachers and some of his class. We had been thrilled that he would have the opportunity as, although Chris and I had looked round the school several times, before the pandemic, Oscar hadn't seen it yet. He'd been a little shy initially, but then suddenly, he'd looked so confident, started interacting with the other kids and listened to the teachers and their instructions. We'd had a tour of the gardens, met some of the animals they kept on site (a pig, chickens and rabbits – which he'd loved), then we'd gone to the forest-school area where they'd all played for a while, before heading to the playground, then inside to see his new classroom.

I knew it was early days, but it made me so emotional (in a good way) to see him so happy there. The anxiety and worry that comes with choosing a new school for any child is huge, but for a child with extra needs, I believe there's a greater responsibility to get it right for them. And that's not taking away all his current school had done for him over the last few years – the teachers, the TAs and the lovely friends he'd made there had been amazing, but if I'm truly honest with myself, Oscar didn't seem as happy at school as he'd once been. I couldn't put my finger on it, but during the months he had had in school leading up to lockdown, he hadn't seemed his usual bubbly self there. It had been obvious that the gap was widening between him and his peers, not just from an academic point of view but from a friendship-forming one. The children had time for him to say hello and maybe involve him in a football game, but I could see they'd lost a bit of interest. After all when you're seven years old and someone can't answer you, it must be frustrating.

But watching Oscar, at what was to be his new school; watching him with teachers who knew their field and understood him and his needs; watching him interact with other children like him, who didn't see 'difference', for the first time in a long time – because, of course, you always doubt the decisions you make on behalf of your kids, don't you? – I got this overwhelming feeling that he would be all right after all. He had been so confident and so happy that day that he'd made me so proud.

At the beginning of July, after a phone call with Oscar's cardiologist talking through the risks of Oscar going back to school versus the risk of his mental health taking a serious knock by staying home for months on end, we made the decision together that, on the grounds of his having an EHCP, he should go back (children who had an EHCP at this point were allowed back in school). It was a tough decision as there were obvious infection risks, but equally Oscar's behaviour at home had been getting increasingly destructive. He needed some focus back, but mostly, whilst the other two were taking it all in their stride, Oscar at this stage just seemed a bit sad now. So, he'd been fortunate enough to be able to attend school for the final three weeks of his final term there, something we will always look back on and be grateful for.

I'd worn sunglasses on Oscar's final day at infant school (thankfully, it was sunny) because I felt sure that it would be emotional. And although it was – he'd been there for the past four years with the most supportive and brilliant faculty and peers – I managed to hold it together. Just about.

And although I knew in my heart of hearts that making the switch from mainstream to SEN was the right move for us now, I couldn't help but feel a pang of sadness, leaving behind so many lovely friends and wonderful teachers and TAs we'd met along the way.

Dear Headteacher, Teachers, TAs and Staff

As Oscar's time at school comes to an end, Chris and I wanted to send you our heartfelt thanks for all you have done for him over the years. If we could thank each one of you personally, we would, for we know, that even if you haven't worked with Oscar directly, you have played a massive part in his time at school. Entrusting any child into the care of a setting is a big deal, but for a parent of a child who has additional needs, the prospect feels all the more daunting. And although Oscar doesn't have the verbal communication to tell us, we KNOW he loved school – and we credit you all for that.

For us it was only ever about our little boy feeling nurtured, wanted and included. We wanted him to have this time with his brother and sister, to work alongside his mainstream peers and feel a sense of belonging. And although we have a long way to go as far as academia is concerned, he has learnt so much from you and all the gorgeous children you teach. So, Thank You for the kindness you have shown him. For the differentiation and the slower pace and for your patience and your understanding. All too often others see a person's diagnosis over and above everything else about them. Thank you for always seeing Oscar first.

Wishing you all a well-deserved break this summer. Stay safe.

Sarah and Chris Roberts

And just like that, the next chapter awaits.

* * * *

We were at a local park and three little girls, about eight or nine years old, started playing 'Lava Monster' with Oscar, Alfie and Flo. It had all been going well and everyone appeared to be having fun, until I noticed one of the girls pulling another away. They then stood whispering to one another. Initially, I couldn't hear what was being said, but they were very obviously looking over at Oscar, so it was very apparent who they'd been talking about. The only thing I heard was one of the girls asking the other girl, 'Because his eyes look funny?', and she'd answered, 'Yes.'

They then made their excuses and left.

And here's the thing, you'd think after all this time, on the very rare occasions when something like this is said (and it really is rare because usually kids are fab), you'd think that it wouldn't affect me. But still, eight years on, I felt the pang. You know, the one that gets you right in the pit of your stomach? And I know what you'll say, they're just kids, they weren't being overtly nasty to his face etc. etc., but it got me thinking about why it made me feel this way.

Oz didn't have a clue. Neither did Alfie or Flo, but I knew first-hand that had they noticed, they too would have felt protective over their brother and that only made me want to protect them all from things like this. I'll be the first to admit that when everyone first started talking about #blacklivesmatter, I had never spoken to my kids about race, believing that because they didn't SEE or acknowledge 'difference' with regard to the colour of a person's skin, I didn't need to. I now realise it's so important we talk to our kids. And I think perhaps this meeting in the park highlighted that again for me, the need to remind us that as parents it's our responsibility to educate our children. On race, on religion AND on disability and how discriminatory it can be, even in somewhere as innocent as a children's playground.

Back in February, Oscar had had a hearing test and it was found that his hearing had deteriorated significantly.

So much so, that having toyed with the idea of more grommets (a procedure that helps a lot of children with their hearing, but unfortunately for Oscar, they never really stayed put) we'd discussed with his ENT consultant the benefits of getting him fitted for hearing aids. The previous day, however, Oscar had had another hearing test. They'd found he had congestion in one ear and a lingering ear infection in the other. Yet, despite this, he managed to smash his hearing test, so much so that they found that his hearing was within normal range. Yet again we were being told he didn't need hearing aids after all. I mean, I've said it before, but this parenting lark really is a rollercoaster, hey? The next day would be the first day at his new school for Oscar and, as I had predicted, panic (mine, not his) had set in.

Blog Comments

'My twins with DS attend specialist school. Our local authority placed them there (they decide placement locations for any child requiring enhanced provision – we are not permitted to name a school or setting). I had worked and volunteered with children with additional needs locally for many years who had attended both mainstream and specialist schools. I also had peers with additional needs, including DS, when I was at primary and high school. I was all too aware of social isolation or superficial friendships in mainstream environments, and the education I had observed was far from inclusive. Our mainstream school visits prior to panel included me being shown separate dinner tables and areas of the

---

playground etc. If I could pause time and sort out all the attitudinal barriers, upskill staff in inclusive education and assistive technology, and more, ready for a school to receive my children then I would have done – we all have the same aspirations for our kids to go to school in our local community with kids with all abilities. Where the schools are not ready to receive, include, and educate children with disabilities, however, the children are the ones that suffer. It isn't about parents and our wants and wishes. It isn't about the experience of other kids in the school. It is about the experience for the child at the centre of it. It is about how they are included, how they are taught, how they are nurtured and how they are respected. It is those factors that, in my opinion, should determine a school placement, whatever the label. It is about balancing the work to be done and the experience of the child. Tweaks, sure. Entire overhauls and blind faith, not so much.

I've been confronted countless times for my boys being in specialist school. I've been asked why I've ignored research, why I don't want my kids to be independent in the future, and why I want to hide them from society. The questions are ignorant, offensive, and the implications are so far from the truth, it's unreal. My boys are academically and socially thriving. They have very bright futures ahead of them. Nobody knows what the future of their child would be if they were in the opposite setting, whether it would be better, the same or worse. Many factors are at play.

I've often felt that many within the DS community who have confronted me about this would be happier if my boys were at mainstream even if they had no friends and had a terrible teaching experience to be honest. Someone once messaged me to berate me for their school placement and included the line "your boys should be in mainstream. End of." Let that sink in. . .'

Elaine Scougal @ollieandcameron

21

Four Myths About Down Syndrome

'Trust that an ending is followed by a beginning'
Unknown

Would he get on the minibus the following morning? (Oscar's new school was approximately forty minutes away and a trip he would have to make without me, on a minibus, with a group of older kids, a driver and an escort.)

Had it registered that he would be going to a NEW school and not the one he'd been at for the past four years?

Would his teachers understand what he wanted when he tried to speak and sign to them?

Would he tell them when he needed the toilet, or leave it until it was way too late?

Would he make new friends?

Would his teachers and peers love him, the way we all do?

Those had been the questions whirling around my head in the early hours of the morning before he started. Oscar had woken, he'd drifted back off quickly, but when I'd usually have no trouble going back to sleep myself, I had laid there feeling anxious. I knew it was normal for any parent to feel worried about their child and the next step. But when you have a child with additional needs, who can't always vocalise what they're thinking and feeling, entrusting them into the care of others, not having that interaction at the school gate any more, embarking on new routines and a new normal. . . it was a massive deal. And I knew we'd done all we could. He seemed excited (he was desperate to put on his new uniform when the other two had headed back to school the day before). We'd put together social stories, he'd had a settling-in session a few months ago, we'd met his escort who'd be with him on his minibus, not to mention emails and calls, filling the school in with all the info they might need. I had been so very certain we were doing the right thing. But, still, new starts are tough.

He was so ready, though. I was SO ready (I couldn't wait for the silence), but I held him a little tighter that evening, mostly because I felt like I needed it, way more than he did.

First day done. As Oscar caught sight of his new minibus pulling into our driveway for the first time, I thought he was about to have a wobble. He looked so unsure initially, but literally seconds afterwards, he practically skipped onto the bus. I don't think he could believe his luck.

In fact, we didn't even manage to get a decent photo of him in his school uniform before he left because he was SO excited from the moment he'd woken up that morning and wouldn't stand still long enough. And having read the write-up in his communication book, it sounded as though he'd had a great first day. So, all in all, a resounding success. You'll be pleased to hear that I managed to hold it together all day too, with just a little blub as the minibus pulled away. Not because I was sad, but because I was just so chuffed. For him.

We'd never made too much of a big deal about Oscar having Down syndrome. To Alfie and Flo, Oscar's just their brother. Like most siblings across the land, they love and infuriate one another, in equal measure. Up until then, we'd always been led by them and the questions they'd just dropped into conversation. But no matter how many times you think you've reiterated that Oz just takes a bit longer to learn stuff, no matter how many times you think they've fully understood, one of them will drop in something, out of nowhere. A while ago now, I spoke about the time Alfie asked me outright if 'Oscar had lost his voice'. It had been one of those situations where, for a few seconds, I'd been completely floored. It was probably the question, though, that originally prompted us to talk to Alfie and Flo about Oscar's diagnosis and what it meant.

We'd had that conversation over a year ago now, but then recently, after a couple of other questions from both Alfie and Flo, e.g. 'Why does Mrs <insert name here> follow Oscar around at school?', 'Will Oscar ever FIND his voice, Mummy?' and, more recently, 'But why does Oscar go to that school and not the big school round the corner?' it got me thinking about these sorts of questions and when (because undoubtedly they will) more come up, how we'd handle answering them.

I think for me, honesty has always been the best policy. Often though, I guess because they were still quite young, they could ask something big, like the time Flo asked me,

'Will Oscar be a daddy first, then Alfie and then me be a mummy?', that left me searching for the right thing to say as a response, but before I had, they'd moved on to the next subject.

I guess I focused on Oscar's potential to achieve – I'd told them he was going to a new school because they would be able to help him achieve X, Y and Z. We answer our kids' questions with as much information as they can understand and I always make sure that the basis of everything is that it sometimes takes Oscar longer to master milestones, but that he gets there in the end. Having Alfie and Flo in his life has meant that Oz is equipped with two of the very best teachers. They unknowingly show him the way and having the three of them so close in age, has just been the best thing for all of them.

*　*　*　*

There are so many myths flying around about DS. Misconceptions, preconceived ideas etc. But our community (that's those that advocate for people who happen to have DS) are very passionate about dispelling those myths and so, with that in mind, here's a little insight into my world with Oscar.

It was around 3 p.m. on a Sunday afternoon and Oscar, Flo and I had been in Marks & Spencer's. Oscar, true to his athletic form, decided that instead of heading to the kid's department on the ground floor, he would instead leg it to the first, via the escalator. The only thing was that he'd decided to go up the wrong escalator, the one most prefer to travel down on, so was now running against the moving stairs, like something out of *Ninja Warrior UK*.

(Myth 1 – People with DS aren't physically able #lies)

Unsure of the best course of action, I waited at the bottom for him to get tired, stop running and make his way down, only of course he didn't get tired because this kid is a machine. So, there I was, standing at the bottom watching most of Marks & Spencer's now watching him. Various people had started down the escalator, realised there was a small child trying to come at them and, rightly so, jumped out of the way of said oncoming boy! Feeling exasperated, I decided to head up the escalator (the one that we were meant to use for going up), only when he saw me approaching the top, ready to come down and meet him on the other one, THAT was the moment he decided to give in and start running down the escalator.

(Myth 2 – People who happen to have DS aren't very clever #begtodiffer)

Cue another five minutes of Flo and me chasing him up and down the escalator, all the while, out of the corner of my eye, I could see and hear the onlooking public gasping in disbelief ('He's going to fall', 'Oh, my!' etc. etc.) I did, however, foil him in the end, though. As he was coming up the escalator I hid behind a display board and jumped out just as he reached the top and grabbed him (much to his amusement). Flo also obviously found this hilarious.

(Myth 3 – Siblings will resent the child who has additional needs and not want to be around them #sheloveshimsomuch)

And I guess, in hindsight, it *was* funny, though perhaps more so if you're not the one chasing him. Oh, and if he hadn't then dropped to the ground and refused to move because he was SO cross with me that his game was now over.

(Myth 4 – Everyone with DS is SO happy all the time)

So here endeth the myth-busting lesson.

* * * *

I'd woken up not feeling it. Oscar had had a dental appointment booked in, which was the first one since being referred to see a specialist SEN dentist and, knowing him the way I did, I wasn't feeling that confident it was going to go well. I'd also had a call from Guy's and St Thomas' hospital in London, to book him in for an overnight sleep study the following week, and whereas I'd usually be pretty upbeat when it came to some of the challenges Oz has to face, sometimes I'd find myself wishing things were simpler.

We'd arrived at the SEN dentist, had our temperatures taken, our hands sanitised and been met by a lovely dental nurse dressed in PPE. She'd been so engaging, had taken the time to speak to Oz and whereas he'd usually become anxious, he'd followed her straight in. We'd next met another nurse and his new dentist, who'd then spent around thirty minutes with him, building up his trust, chatting with him and making him laugh a lot. He'd spent the first ten minutes looking out the window. (He'd spotted the dental chair and wasn't having any of that), so they'd stood next to him, commenting on the cars, the houses, asking him about school (all the while, having a sneaky look at his teeth any time he'd opened his mouth). We'd tried him on my lap, but he ended up jumping off and hiding under the table. I was thinking at that point it'd probably be game over, but both the dentist and the nurse then crouched down to chat with him again and eventually they'd both climbed under the table with him, which Oscar thought was hilarious.

I'm not going to say he had a full examination because he didn't. But they had managed to see most of his teeth and at the end of the appointment, so they could build on that trust, the dentist suggested we brought Oscar back in a couple of weeks' time to see her.

As I was driving Oz back to school, I reflected on the appointment and how brilliant they'd been with him. There they'd been, in full PPE, on their hands and knees, under a table, taking the time to really make Oscar feel safe. Times were tough for so many, but that visit really restored my faith in just how gorgeous people could be with kids like Oscar. It was an example of people showing true kindness and taking the time. Kindness and your time – two of the most important things you can give a person.

* * * *

A few years ago, when I'd been presenting a talk to a group of doctors, I'd explained to them where 'Don't Be Sorry' (the name of my social media page) had come from. I told them that shortly after Oscar had been born and when we were told by his paediatrician the unexpected news that he had Down syndrome, she had started her sentence with an apology. And although her words have always stayed with me – 'I'm so sorry, but we suspect your baby has Down syndrome' – I've often thought back to the way she made us feel that night and the impact of her reaction to our news.

When I'd explained this to this group of doctors, one of them had raised his hand. He'd challenged me by saying that he too would have said much the same, because that was what they'd been taught in medical school. He then went on to say that whenever they got to deliver news, in his words, 'like cancer or a tumour' they'd been told to say sorry. On my drive home that day I remember being annoyed with myself that I hadn't challenged him, because whilst I understood cancer or a tumour to be illnesses and therefore something one might feel sorry about having, who had he been to assume that Down syndrome, a condition, not an illness, should be regarded in the same light as cancer?

The day after the trip to the dentist, I received a letter in the post from one of Oscar's consultants. And under the subheading PROBLEMS, the first thing listed was Trisomy 21 (Down syndrome) and I couldn't help feeling that we still had so far to go. To his consultant, Trisomy 21 may have felt like a 'problem'. Perhaps to the outside world and to anyone who hadn't had experience themselves, Oscar's diagnosis may have looked like a problem to them too? But to reiterate (because I know I've said all this many times before), our words are so important. Each word that we use has an impact. A word at first glance may seem inconsequential. But the words we choose, both professionally and personally, have the power to change things, for better or worse.

A few weeks later, I was asked to give a presentation to seventy doctors, all of whom are on the GPVTS (GP Vocational Training Scheme) at Coventry and Warwickshire Hospital. It would be the third year that I'd presented there, although this time, it was over Zoom. The brief was 'A parent's perspective'. So I spoke about Oscar's birth and his subsequent diagnosis. I talked about the paediatrician's apology and the negative language used. I told them I now realised their unconscious bias played a big part in how they saw my newborn son and the preconceived idea they had about the life he'd go on to lead. I told them that I knew that when people met Oscar, they often saw his diagnosis first, before they truly saw *him*. But I let them know that, in my opinion, Oscar wasn't defined by his condition. He wasn't a 'Down's boy', he was Oscar. . . who just happens to have Down syndrome.

I'd spoken about the language used around screening for Down syndrome and how when giving women their results, using 'chance' or 'likelihood' sounded so much better than 'risk'. The word 'risk' is something that exposes you to danger, which is the very last thing Oscar has exposed me to.

I told them about the letters we'd all received from GP surgeries and hospitals, listing DS under the subheading 'Problems'. And how making a small amendment to their master document and switching it to 'Diagnosis' or 'Condition' is all it would take. I said more. A lot more. I told them I have the utmost respect and appreciation for the job they do and that I would be forever grateful for the continued care Oscar receives. But I hope that hearing from me made them stop and think about the lasting impression our words have.

I believe we're all wearing lenses, in the way we see the world and I think the more aware we are, and the better we know where our prejudices lie, the better. As a counsellor in training, it's about being open to conversations and acknowledging that the assumptions we make about a person shape the way we hear a person's story. It's a big ask and we still have a long way to go, but I hope people are always open to learning more about someone like Oscar, I really do.

I was contacted by a woman the other day, who said that although she knew her five-year-old (who had DS) needed to get out, when they did, they wouldn't walk or go in the wheelchair. Then once they'd decided they would walk again they'd kept running off. We'd had this for so many years with Oscar. And although on the odd occasion, he would still bolt, he didn't do it as much as before and we had learnt over the years what Oscar's triggers were.

It may sound ridiculous to any other parent of an eight- or nine-year-old, because when they're that bit older, you do tend to trust that your kid won't do anything unpredictable, but for every second I'd been out with Oscar, I had been trying to pre-empt what he might do; I was ready to react. We'd gone on a walk with friends, and he'd been as good as gold, but I knew from the moment we'd stepped out of the car that there was always a chance that he would run off. I put him in wellies (to slow him down) and felt pleased that he'd spent most of the walk collecting stones and rocks that he'd place in his pockets or carry, which would, again, slow him right down.

Our house is now Oscar-proofed. We have locks in the top corner of every door upstairs, so that when we're not in them, we can lock them behind us and keep Oz out. If we left them open, he would literally turn the room over. We have locks on the fridge and cupboards otherwise he'd spend every moment of the school holidays helping himself to snacks!!!! But things have got easier. And I think it's a mix of Oscar growing up – he loves sticking with the gang if we are out with Alfie and Flo or other kids, so doesn't tend to run off, but we've also probably got a bit wiser as to what works for us.

My social media pages and books have never been about dishing out advice, more about solidarity and finding comfort in knowing that someone else gets it. Just because I write about Oscar and our experiences doesn't mean this is how it's going to be for every child who happens to have DS. Each child is a unique individual, who may struggle in some areas in which others don't. Equally, some excel in areas that others find harder. There isn't a one-size-fits-all approach.

Blog Comments

'For me I selected the local mainstream school for several reasons. . . His older brother was there; there was already a student with DS we knew there; they were positive about taking him (and his bestie Ella!); it was part of the community; it was easier logistics; I was close to support. But now looking at secondary options I'm torn with no option looking ideal/available to us!'

@themathsmum

'My son Adam went to our local mainstream school and moved to a SEN school for secondary. In retrospect I wish he had transitioned in Year 5 when the TAs found it too difficult to adapt and keep him involved in the class. For Adam SEN school has been the making of him and has certainly taken the pressure off me as a parent as I always felt as though I was the one educating the teachers how best to teach a child with Down syndrome. At the end of the day, it all depends on the individual child, the school's ability to give your child the best opportunities to fulfil their potential. Adam is having his eighteenth birthday party tonight with friends coming from his mainstream primary and his SEN friends.'

@juliaryan43

'I'm in a constant state of turmoil around what is best and feel really torn! There is no solid advice, informative decision-making processes or guides. I genuinely feel in our situation it's luck of the draw in terms of how inclusive, receptive and open to making "reasonable adjustments" (we all love that term!) a mainstream school is, coupled with the teachers and 1-2-1s you luck out getting! Hence my thoughts on this change annually depending on that. Ultimately, it's ludicrous that my child's progress in school and ability to fulfil his potential is based on luck and those around him at a particular time. But the decision is so final. . . I wish there were more split placements. . . so you get the best mix of both dependent on the child.'

@t21teamkush

22

'Oscar's Awesome'

*'In three words I can sum up everything
I've learned about life – It. Goes. On.'*
Robert Frost

I was hesitant initially to write about Oscar and how things
have been going, as far as him transitioning to his new
school is concerned. Mainly because I didn't want to gush
too much, for fear of it all going wrong. This time round it
has been quite different because there has been literally no
face-to-face contact with his teacher or TAs. You don't see
them at the door when your child is dismissed after school
any more and when you might once have got a reassuring
thumbs up or a smile, letting you know they'd done okay
that day (or the chance to discuss any issues that might have
come up), instead he now heads off every morning on his
minibus, comes home that way too and the only feedback
we've had so far has been via his communication book and
the secure online portal where his teacher posts a photo or
comment and we can write a response.

Oscar has never been able to tell us what he's been up
to at school, in so much as he hasn't ever had the words.

Early in his first term, when he got a certificate for being 'Star Player' in football and another for 'Good listening and following instructions', he'd come bounding through the front door and gone straight to his bag to pull out his certificates to show us. He'd been so happy with himself.

And that's how we felt. There'd been a shift and he seemed SO happy. The communication we had via the book had been nothing but positive. There was a real sense that the people working with him genuinely loved their jobs. I suppose it was that thing, that they've chosen to work with children like Oscar and others like him and their positivity and enthusiasm shone through. Nothing seemed too much trouble. There had always been a part of me that had been worrying every single day Oscar had been at his last school – wondering if he'd been behaving; if he'd been compliant; if he'd been involved enough; if he'd had a toileting accident; was it all too much of a hindrance to them. . . I guess, ultimately, had he been too much? It was only now that he was settling in to his new school that I felt this real sense of calm. And that was the case for both of us.

We did have one minor blip when he first started, in that he managed somehow to set the fire alarm off. When I received the phone call about it, I held my breath, thinking they were going to tell me they didn't want him any more because he was too much of a nightmare. I know I have a habit of catastrophising things, but I think any SEN parent can vouch for me when I say that often we worry that our kids are causing too much trouble. I needn't have worried though; the teacher was so lovely about it and said that he wasn't the first, wouldn't be the last and that it was the school's fault for having the alarms set so low for little hands to touch. I put the phone down and felt this huge sense of relief. The way they'd spoken about Oscar was with genuine affection and fondness and it was at that moment that I realised, he was exactly where he needed to be.

Oscar's little face would light up when we spoke about school together, which is all any parent could ask for. So, I am going to go out on a limb here and say, it is going well. He is happy and we are so very proud of how he's handling it all.

* * * *

Towards the end of the first term at his new school, I had had a lovely follow-up call from a professional who works with Oscar. She had visited him in his previous school and has since observed him in his new setting. She's spoken about how she felt emotional seeing him in his new setting. How (and this is no disrespect to his previous school) it was 'like night and day' and that he'd 'found his tribe'. She said he was engaged in activities in the classroom setting and he just looked so happy. We've had feedback from the school, and we've seen the change in Oscar for ourselves, but hearing positives from an outsider made it more special and I had tears in my eyes as I hung up the phone.

Something I touched on earlier and which perhaps concludes this tale, for now at least, is what Oscar has brought me by way of self-development. If you'd told me the day he was born that having him would lead me here, I wouldn't have believed you for a second. By sharing his life online, writing books and public speaking, I have found myself on a very different path to the one I imagined when I first fell pregnant with him and the subsequent, different one I imagined I'd be on as a 'special needs mum'. I have openly said that having Oscar has its challenges, but over and above all that, being Oscar's mummy has opened my eyes up to so many more opportunities than I ever imagined. In September 2020, I decided to take a leap of faith and sign up to a course to become a counselling psychotherapist. Over the years, listening to others talk about their experiences – their low moments, their worries, their fears – I realised I was making a difference by giving them the space to talk openly and honestly without passing judgement. I too understood the benefits of sharing my own anxieties and how opening up about them helps immensely. Over time I realised that whatever our circumstances, whatever life throws at us, we all have the capacity to turn things around, if we want to. And although it is easier for some than for others, we all have choices about the way we look at and deal with things, and I want now to help others see that, like me, they can keep moving forwards. So, I signed up to the course. And having not studied anything since 1999 (and even that was with my feet), it feels so good to be learning again. I'm loving the potential for new beginnings, and I love that my darling boy has given me the drive and ambition to do all this. If all goes to plan, by June 2023, I will be a fully qualified psychotherapist, and I cannot wait to start.

Last summer, just as Oscar turned nine, we went camping. We'd attempted camping a couple of years before, but it had all felt like a lot of effort for just one night away. It also felt a lot as far as Oscar was concerned. Back then we'd just started properly toilet training him. I'd had my egg-timer that went off every thirty minutes in the hope that he'd 'perform' on the loo, but it was disastrous. We'd also had to follow him around everywhere because we couldn't trust that he'd stay close by and I remember feeling so on edge the whole time, worrying he'd wander off.

This time, we did two nights away and it dawned on me whilst there that Oscar was different this year. When he

went out of sight for a few moments, we knew he'd stay
with the other children we'd gone with. He joined in the
games, he loved helping with some of the camping duties
and I'd loved watching him as he got involved.

I remember wondering a few years ago if we'd ever get
out of the running-off phase. If I'm truly honest, there were
times I'd felt cheesed off that I was the one still shadowing
my child so closely, whilst others with kids the same
age were sitting chatting, without the need to worry. I'd
wondered then if we'd ever be able to sit by the campfire
and relax with our friends. And whilst I will forever keep
one eye out, because, let's face it, he's an opportunist and
I'm not THAT stupid, this camping trip felt closer to what
everyone else experiences. We even managed to sit around
the campfire with a gin in a tin.

Just as we were leaving, one of our camp mates, who'd
been a friend of a friend and who'd never met Oz before,
stood watching him playing with the other kids and turned
to me and said, 'Oscar's awesome.'

When people have said that in the past, I might have
agreed, but offered the caveat, 'But he's a handful,' but this
time, I didn't. I just agreed. Because he really is.

As Oscar's mum, every once in a while people will say
to me: 'I don't know how you do it, I don't think I could.'

It's a phrase, or something along those lines, that I've
heard many, many times since Oscar was born.

It's not a phrase I take exception to, as I know it's coming
from a good place and those who say it are doing so to
show their support. But sometimes, rather than smiling or
shrugging it off, here's what I'd ACTUALLY like to say:

'When your son is taking a little longer to reach each
milestone and you feel deflated at times because he's
lagging, I promise you, you could do it.

251

'When your child is playing in the park and you spend your time shadowing him rather than standing talking to your friends, where I'm pretty sure all the other mums and dads of boys his age are standing, I'm sure you could do it.

'When your son wakes you up throughout the night for the fourth week in a row because he has recurring ear infections or the heaviest cold, even though you have never felt so exhausted in your entire life, I bet you could do it.

'When you get yet another appointment letter through the door asking you to take him to see another consultant/doctor/therapist, you might sigh because you feel a bit gutted for him (and for yourself), but I promise you, you could do it.

'And when he wakes every single morning before the sun comes up, no matter how tired you're feeling, I KNOW you could do it.

'For every hour longer you spend reminding him how to do something, how to behave, how to become the young man he so desperately wants to become, you are reminded in moments like this, of exactly HOW you do it.

'And it won't be because you *must*, and it won't be because it's a chore, it'll be because, when all's said and done, he's yours and you love him with your full heart.'

So, when someone says, 'I don't know how you do it, I don't think I could.' My reply would be simply, 'You could, and I promise you, you absolutely would.'